Interacting with Patients

Interacting with Patients

Joyce Samhammer Hays, B.S., M.S., R.N.

Consultant in Psychiatric Nursing, Veterans Administration Hospitals. Northport, Long Island, and Perry Point, Maryland; formerly Director of the Psychiatric Nursing Program, School of Nursing, University of Pennsylvania, Philadelphia.

Kenneth H. Larson, B.S., R.N.

Associate Director of Nurses, Psychiatric Division, Bellevue Hospital Center, New York; formerly Clinical Supervisor, Nursing Service, Veterans Administration Hospital, Northport, Long Island

The Macmillan Company, New York

Collier-Macmillan Limited, London

Seventh Printing, 1969

Library of Congress catalog card number: 63–13572

The Macmillan Company, New York
Collier-Macmillan Canada, Ltd., Toronto, Ontario

Printed in the United States of America

To Janesy B. Myers
whose support and encouragement
were invaluable and unlimited

Foreword

IN 1926 A PROMINENT PSYCHIATRIST SUGGESTED THAT NURSES WORKING in psychiatric facilities secure for themselves "a well-trained technic." Since then, nurses have slowly been evolving and defining aspects of a "technic." Simple, clear guidelines are greatly needed, particularly to guide the verbal exchanges that nursing personnel have with patients. The pathology of the patient is often more evident in his verbal behavior than in gross actions; further, constructive intervention is mediated through the verbal exchange of nurse with patient. So this aspect of nursing practice is most important. This book will help clarify for the nurse various dimensions of the verbal exchanges that she has with patients.

What the nurse says to a patient can be variously classified. The nurse can make a spontaneous comment—reacting verbally with the first idea that comes to mind in response to the patient's behavior. The nurse can make a stereotyped, automatic comment—using clichés that are popular in society, or in the hospital subculture, and that serve the main purpose of saying "something" rather than something specific to the patient. The nurse's comments can be grounded in theory—concepts held in the mind of the nurse which help her to explain to herself what the patient may be saying and which guide her choice of words to use in reacting to the patient. Similarly, the nurse can use general principles that guide her verbal comments. Such principles can be stated and studied in advance, so that a rationale for their usage can be considered and understood as a basis for conscious behavior on the part of the nurse.

The authors of this book have taken the nurse-patient relationship apart and scrutinized carefully the various techniques that are used in nurse-patient interactions. Then, they have defined these techniques and illustrated them for the purposes of helping other nursing personnel to achieve similar understanding. This is a valuable effort that ought certainly to speed up efforts within the nursing profession to evolve "a well-trained technic."

This work can be looked upon as a beginning procedure manual for psychiatric units. In the general hospital the technical procedures are generally outlined in such a manual, but these are of so concrete a nature that even pictures can be used to illustrate a particular technique. In psychiatric work, however, the "technical procedures" are more esoteric; this is because of the considerable abstractness in psychiatric work. A picture cannot be painted of a nurse-patient interaction except in words. Similarly, the interpersonal techniques can be conveyed only through word descriptions; and their usage in clinical situations must be conceptualized individually. That is, each nurse must see for herself the relation between the behavior of the patient and the particular interpersonal technique the nurse is using. It is this abstractness in psychiatric work that makes the work difficult and that has slowed up developments in the field; it is easier to talk about a "nursing arts procedure" than it is to talk with definiteness about an interpersonal procedure. Yet, it is necessary as nursing moves toward full professional status that nurses define interpersonal procedures that are found to be useful in nursing practice. This book is a constructive step in this direction.

A professional person ought to have a wide range of technical and interpersonal procedures readily available to recall and use as the work situation requires them. Not only should the professional person be able to use them but also, more importantly, the professional worker should be able to say what procedures are being used at a given moment. Consciousness of usage of interpersonal procedure (the same can be said for theory) is a goal of all students of nursing practices. In order to achieve awareness of this kind, it is first necessary to be fully familiar with various aspects of each interpersonal procedure, to test out its use in clinical practice, to gradually revise one's conceptions so that the procedure is clearly known in relation to the problematic situations in which it serves useful purposes. This book, which derives from the clinical practices observed or carried out by the authors, is a first work that promises considerable assistance to nurse practitioners in achieving consciousness of the interpersonal techniques that they use in relationships with patients.

HILDEGARD E. PEPLAU, R.N., Ed.D.
Professor of Nursing,
Director, Graduate Program in
Advanced Psychiatric Nursing
Rutgers, the State University of
New Jersey

Preface

THE NURSE OF TODAY IS NOT ONLY A SKILLED TECHNICIAN, BUT ALSO she has a broad base of scientific and medical knowledge. She is prepared to manage a complex ward, supervise other personnel, handle effectively a wide variety of emergency situations, and assist the physician in any number of difficult medical and surgical procedures. But, too frequently, she receives very little preparation in another important function: talking with patients. When it is of a therapeutic and constructive nature, verbal interaction is one of the nurse's primary tools in meeting the patient's emotional needs. For every sick person is more than physically ill; he is also anxious, perhaps fearful or angry, sometimes even severely depressed or disturbed. Obviously, emotional problems are not confined solely to the realm of the psychiatric hospital. Hence, *every* nurse—irrespective of the setting in which she functions—has the responsibility of caring for the *whole* person who is the patient. To meet only his physical needs is to care for merely a part of him.

Moreover, the nurse is asking and seeking to learn to interact therapeutically with patients. She wants to know what she can say to the patient whom she is preparing for surgery; the child who is separated from his mother; the patient who is incurably ill or who is dying; the woman in labor; the demanding patients; and the quiet ones who never ask for anything. It is to nurses who must cope with these problems as well as to those who work with psychiatric patients that this work is directed. There are no answers here, but there are guiding principles.

The authors wish to acknowledge their indebtedness to the many members of the nursing staff of the Veterans Administration Hospital, Northport, Long Island, New York, whose work with patients and discussion of problems contributed to the authors' thinking; to Dr. Arnold A. Schillinger, Hospital Director, and Dr. Angelo D. Carra, Chief of Staff, for permission to carry through this work; and especially to Janesy B. Myers, Chief, Nursing

Service, for providing the kind of democratic nursing milieu in which both the authors and the work were able to grow.

The authors also acknowledge their gratitude to Hildegard E. Peplau, Professor of Nursing and Director, Advanced Program in Psychiatric Nursing, College of Nursing, Rutgers—The State University of New Jersey, who not only read much of the manuscript and offered many valuable suggestions, but whose teachings, writings, and theoretical formulations are so much a part of this work.

The management and staff of the Veterans Administration Hospital, Coatesville, Pennsylvania, also deserve the authors' thanks, since much of the early clinical material was gathered there.

Appreciation is also expressed to Ruth Spangler, Instructor in Psychiatric Nursing, School of Nursing, University of Pennsylvania, Philadelphia, and to Harriet Hernandez, Instructor in Pediatric Nursing, Albert Einstein Medical Center, Northern Division, Philadelphia, for supervising the collection of additional clinical material by student nurses.

Finally the authors wish to extend their thanks to their instructors, colleagues, students, and patients—all of whom are represented in this work.

J. S. H.
K. L.

Contents

Foreword vii

Preface ix

Introduction 1

I. INTERPERSONAL TECHNIQUES

Therapeutic 7

Using Silence; Accepting; Giving Recognition; Offering Self; Giving Broad Openings; Offering General Leads; Placing the Event in Time or in Sequence; Making Observations; Encouraging Description of Perceptions; Encouraging Comparison; Restating; Reflecting; Focusing; Exploring; Giving Information; Seeking Clarification; Presenting Reality; Voicing Doubt; Seeking Consensual Validation; Verbalizing the Implied; Encouraging Evaluation; Attempting to Translate into Feelings; Suggesting Collaboration; Summarizing; Encouraging Formulation of a Plan of Action

Nontherapeutic 24

Reassuring; Giving Approval; Rejecting; Disapproving; Agreeing; Disagreeing; Advising; Probing; Challenging; Testing; Defending; Requesting an Explanation; Indicating the Existence of an External Source; Belittling Feelings Expressed; Making Stereotyped Comments; Giving Literal Responses; Using Denial; Interpreting; Introducing an Unrelated Topic

II. ILLUSTRATIVE CLINICAL MATERIAL

Study 1. Mr. John H. 41
A Relationship with a Hostile Patient

Study 2. Mr. V. 65
First Hour of a Nurse-patient Relationship

Study 3. Mr. Karl C. 70
A Relationship with a Suicidal Patient

Study 4. Mr. W. B. 90
Excerpts from a Nurse-patient Relationship

Study 5. Mr. Frank D. 94
Excerpts from a Nurse-patient Relationship

Study 6. Mr. F. E. 99
An Hour with an Autistic Patient

Study 7. Tommy M. 103
Interaction on a Pediatric Unit

Study 8. Johnny S. 105
Interaction on a Pediatric Unit

Study 9. Mr. Joseph W. 109
A Neurologic Patient

Study 10. Mrs. A. F. 113
Relating to the Patient in Labor

Study 11. Mrs. P. 115
Excerpts from a Delivery Room Discussion Immediately Postpartum

Study 12. Mrs. L. 117
Interaction with a New Mother

Study 13. Mrs. J. 119

Excerpts from a Discussion with a Surgical Patient

Study 14. Mr. R. 121

Interaction with a Medical Patient

Study 15. Mr. K. 124

Excerpts from a Discussion with a Patient Admitted for Medical Observation

Study 16. Mr. Fred G. 126

A Relationship with a Patient on an Admission Service

Study 17. Mr. Albert S. 229

A Relationship with a Patient on a Disturbed Unit

Bibliography 275

Index 277

Interacting with

Patients

Introduction

The nurse is recognizing greater opportunities to participate therapeutically with emotionally disturbed persons. These opportunities occur in many settings—in the general hospital, the clinic, the home, the school, in industry, as well as in those settings devoted to psychiatric care. Emphasis is being placed on the nurse's—and other nursing personnel—having more time to spend with those persons in her care. She (or he) is expected to involve herself in direct patient care and to establish therapeutic nurse-patient relationships. Nurses welcome this increased responsibility because they are interested in promoting health. Few nurses, however, have been adequately prepared for this function. The nurse is aware that she should be with patients, listen, express interest, answer questions if possible, and not increase the patients' anxiety. But she is often uncertain of how to proceed beyond these first steps. The best preparation, of course, is a carefully supervised nurse-patient relationship in which the nurse is given expert guidance. It will be some time before any large number of nurses receive such preparation.

To relate therapeutically with a patient it is necessary for the nurse to understand her role and its relationship to the patient's illness. *Emotional illness* is a pattern of living—of thinking, feeling, and behaving—that a person adopts in an attempt to lessen his anxiety and solve his problems in relating to others. Although this way of life reduces anxiety, it does not really solve any problems. It merely postpones problems, while preventing the individual from using his capacities fully and from living a satisfying and productive life. Moreover, this way of living tends to become unacceptable to other people—to members of the individual's family (even though they may participate in it) and to the community as a whole. Hence the patient comes to seek professional help—either because of his own discomfort or through the efforts of others.

A patient enters hospital because he has had severe difficulty in living in the outside world, most frequently in living with other people. . . . for the majority of psychiatric patients, further hospitalization has two functions. One is to protect the patient and those about him from the effects of his illness; the other to provide experiences in living which will enable him to establish relationships that are less anxiety-provoking and more comfortable, thereby making the prospect of further relationships less forbidding. In this latter function, the nurse's role becomes especially meaningful and purposeful, and an integral part of the total regime.

The relationship can be close enough in favourable settings to permit detailed study of a particular patient's special fears, symptoms, or difficulties with others, a detailed study which can be carried out by the nurse and patient, often right in the troublesome situation when it occurs. The nurse can work out difficult incidents with patients precisely because she herself is involved so closely in his ordinary activities. Because of this, her thoughts, feelings, and actions are closely related to the thoughts, feelings, and actions of the patient. A change, or new understanding achieved by her, is likely to bring about a favourable change in the patient's grasp of his problem and the problem itself.

. . . The nurse's contact with patients, extended in time, frequently repeated, intimate in nature, and varied in scope, places her in a unique position to help patients with the personal difficulties in living which they could not solve in the community. Because of this, the third aspect of her functioning—the interpersonal—becomes of central importance: in fact it is the essential part of her task. Interpersonal relations occur during all phases of the patient's life in the hospital—from the most usual events such as eating and sleeping, to the most complex such as participation in the planning of his own living. The therapeutic task of the nurse with the patient will be dependent upon the provision of interpersonal opportunities, both between individuals and in groups, wherein the patient may learn about his problems in living with others, and have help in solving them through more productive experiences.

The nurse must therefore develop the interpersonal skills that enable her to work with patients in these therapeutic experiences.[1]

The *role of the nurse* is to provide the patient with the opportunity (1) to identify and explore his problems in relating to others, (2) to discover healthy ways of meeting his emotional needs, and (3) to experience a satisfying interpersonal relationship. Moreover, it is the nurse's responsibility to make her role explicit to the patient. She cannot expect him to know intuitively why she is there. While sick people tend to see nurses as "helping" persons, such help is usually seen as being provided only in the area of physical comfort and relief from bodily pain. Hence, the nurse must feel free to discuss her role quite openly with the patient so that misconceptions can be cleared away and the nurse-patient relationship utilized fully.

For the nurse to carry out her therapeutic role effectively, she must become aware of the means by which she is interacting with the patient. In this book these means will be referred to as "interpersonal techniques." *Every comment* the nurse makes to the patient (or within his hearing) can be evaluated as having therapeutic or nontherapeutic value; i.e., it either contributes to his emotional growth or it reinforces his illness. Al-

[1] WHO. *Expert Committee on Psychiatric Nursing. First report.* World Health Organization Technical Report Series, No. 105, July 1956.

though the spoken word is focused on here, this applies to nonverbal communication as well. And it applies to comments made to the patient in the course of carrying out other functions, such as giving medications, bathing, assisting with treatments, or even brief, casual contacts, as well as during time set aside for the individual nurse-patient relationship.

While the authors do not propose to suggest a "system" of psychotherapeutic interviewing, it is their aim to present some principles that will be useful—useful in everyday verbal exchanges among patients and nursing personnel as well as in more prolonged counseling relationships.

The purpose of this book is to encourage the nurse, and other members of the nursing team, to evaluate each of her verbal exchanges with patients, determine the techniques she uses most frequently, eliminate nontherapeutic techniques, and learn some additional techniques to aid her in interacting more therapeutically with patients, for if the nurse is not guided by the impulse of the moment, but rather by some explicit and clinically tried principles, her therapeutic impact will be greatly enhanced.

It should be kept in mind, however, that the list of interpersonal techniques described herein is not meant to be exhaustive. Certainly other categories could be added that would be of equal value.

Nor should the techniques in themselves be overvalued. The techniques are tools, not ends in themselves. They are only as therapeutic as the person who employs them. Any single technique—even a therapeutic one—can be used too frequently to have usefulness. For example, for the nurse to utilize only restatement would make her of little value to the patient. The judicious selection of the most appropriate technique must be made at the moment—after the patient has spoken and before the nurse responds. Moreover, just exactly which idea or feeling the nurse selects to restate or clarify or focus upon is more crucial than the particular technique employed. The feelings the nurse has toward the patient and his perceptions of her also play a large part in the relationship.[2]

All things considered, the techniques play only a limited role. But if they serve as a guide, offering the nurse a greater variety of responses to the patient, limiting the frequency of her nontherapeutic utterances, and making her more aware of what it is she is doing as she interacts with patients, this work will have served its purpose.

[2] Rogers, Carl R.: "Characteristics of a Helping Relationship," *Personnel and Guidance Journal* (September 1958) reprinted as Supplement #27, *Canada's Mental Health,* March 1962, pp. 10–15.

I

Interpersonal Techniques

Therapeutic Techniques

1. USING SILENCE . . . utilizing absence of verbal communication.

Silence in itself often encourages the patient to verbalize if it is an interested, expectant silence. This kind of silence indicates to the patient that the nurse expects him to speak, to take the initiative, to communicate that which is most pressing. It gives the patient the opportunity to collect and organize his thoughts, to think through a point, or to consider introducing a topic of greater concern to him than the one being discussed. A positive and accepting silence can be a valuable therapeutic tool. It encourages the patient to talk; directs his thoughts to the task at hand—the consideration of his problem; reduces the pace of the interview when either the nurse or the patient is pressing or pushing too hard; gives the patient time to consider alternative courses of action, delve deeply into his feelings, or weigh a decision; and allows the patient to discover that he can be accepted even though he is silent, that even though he is shy and quiet, he has worth and is respected by another person.[1]

Much nonverbal communication occurs during these interludes. The nurse needs to be alert to what she is communicating as well as perceiving. Even momentary loss of interest can be interpreted as indifference. Schwartz and Shockley[2] state that the utilization of silence is often difficult for nursing personnel, since

> . . . they think that nothing is happening and that they are wasting their time. In long periods of silence, they become bored and their attention wanders from the patient. If the nurse could observe the patient and herself carefully, she might discover that a great deal happens between them at these times.

[1] Brammer, Lawrence M., and Everett L. Shostrom: *Therapeutic Psychology: Fundamentals of Counseling and Psychotherapy*. Englewood Cliffs, N. J.: Prentice-Hall, 1960, pp. 192–93.

[2] Schwartz, Morris S., and Emmy Lanning Shockley: *The Nurse and the Mental Patient*. New York: Russell Sage Foundation, 1956, p. 101.

2. ACCEPTING . . . giving indication of reception.

"Yes."
"Uh hmm."
"I follow what you said."
Nodding.

An accepting response, such as "I'm with you" or "I follow what you're saying," indicates that the nurse has heard and has followed the trend of thought. Such responses signify that the nurse is attuned to the patient, that communication is occurring, and that she is a participant rather than a passive observer. Accepting does not indicate agreement but is non-judgmental in character. "It is simply a verbalization of the attitudes of permissiveness and acceptance of the counselor which say in effect: 'Go on, it's safe, you needn't be ashamed of expressing how you really feel.' "[3]

It should not need to be added that the nurse does not imply that she understands when she does not. Rogers[4] adds,

> Accepting does not mean much until it involves understanding. It is only as I *understand* the feelings and thoughts which seem so horrible to you, or so weak, or so sentimental or so bizarre—it is only as I see them as you see them, and accept them and you, that you can feel really free to explore all the hidden nooks and frightening crannies of your inner and oftentimes buried experience.

Not only the words are important, but also the facial expression, the tone of voice and inflection, and the posture of the nurse. All must convey the same feeling of acceptance.[5] If they do not, the words will be meaningless.

3. GIVING RECOGNITION . . . acknowledging, indicating awareness.

"Good morning, Mr. S."
"You've tooled a leather wallet."
"I notice that you've combed your hair."

To greet the patient by name, to indicate awareness of change, to note the efforts the patient has made—these and other similar indications by the nurse show that she recognizes the patient as a person, as an individual. Such recognition carries with it none of the burden for him that praise or approval imposes. It does not imply that one thing is "good" and its opposite, "bad." Nor does it cause the patient to strive for more and more

[3] Brammer and Shostrom, *op. cit.*, p. 182.
[4] Rogers, Carl R.: "A Counseling Approach to Human Problems," *Am. J. Nursing*, **56**:994–97, August 1956.
[5] Brammer and Shostrom, *op. cit.*, p. 182.

approval for its own sake. Peplau comments quite simply, "When a patient accomplishes something that is a fact, a nurse can say so."[6]

4. OFFERING SELF . . . making one's *self* available.

"I'll sit with you awhile."
"I'll stay here with you."
"I'm interested in your comfort."

The patient may not be ready to communicate verbally with another person. Or the patient may not be able to make himself understood. Often the nurse can offer only her presence, her interest, and her desire to understand. To be therapeutic this offer must be made unconditionally, i.e., without the patient's feeling that he must give in order to receive or that the nurse will stay only if he does or does not do this or that. (However, those conditions that do apply should be stated, e.g., *all* the nurse's time is not available to the patient.) On this point Peplau says, "The patient must deny her own feelings and needs in order to be accepted and liked by a nurse who is *conditional* in her relations with the patient."[7]

5. GIVING BROAD OPENINGS . . . allowing the patient to take the initiative in introducing the topic.

"Is there something you'd like to talk about?"
"What are you thinking about?"
"Where would you like to begin?"

Broad opening comments merely make explicit the idea that the lead is to be taken by the patient. For the patient who is hesitant or uncertain as to what role he is to play in the interaction, these openings, such as "Is there anything you'd like to discuss with me?" stimulate him to take the initiative and to feel that this is what is expected of him. The nurse should avoid the conventional pleasantries when greeting the patient and refrain from making "small talk." If the nurse does start the discussion, she can try to alter this situation by asking, "Would you like to talk about yourself now?" and then waiting silently until the patient takes over.[8]

6. OFFERING GENERAL LEADS . . . giving encouragement to continue.

[6] Peplau, Hildegard E.: *Interpersonal Relations in Nursing.* New York: G. P. Putnam's Sons, 1952, p. 236.
[7] *Ibid.*, p. 185.
[8] Wolberg, Lewis R.: *The Technique of Psychotherapy.* New York: Grune and Stratton, 1954, p. 161.

"Go on."
"And then?"
"Tell me about it."

General leads, such as "And after that?" or "Go on," leave the direction of the discussion almost entirely to the patient. They indicate that the nurse is following what has been said and is interested in what is to come next. Brown and Fowler[9] comment:

> The verbal activity of the nurse is at a minimum with the patient doing most of the talking. The nurse encourages the patient to talk by her nonverbal activity such as nodding or various gestures. If verbal activity becomes necessary, sometimes just a word such as "well" or "really" will enable the patient to continue.

Schwartz and Shockley state that the nurse "waits for" the patient's communication, "goes along with" or follows his leads, and takes the cue from him rather than directing the discussion herself.[10]

7. PLACING THE EVENT IN TIME OR IN SEQUENCE . . . clarifying the relationship of events in time.

"What seemed to lead up to. . . ?"
"Was this before or after. . . ?"
"When did this happen?"

Putting events in their proper sequence helps both the nurse and the patient to see them in perspective. The extent to which one event may have led to another can be viewed more objectively once a certain amount of chronologic ordering has occurred. And at times it will become obvious to the patient that previously accepted cause-and-effect relationships could not exist. The nurse may find that she is then able to identify a recurring pattern of interpersonal difficulties, giving her clues to the kind of satisfying experiences with others that the patient needs.

8. MAKING OBSERVATIONS . . . verbalizing what is perceived.

"You appear tense."
"Are you uncomfortable when you. . . ?"
"I notice that you're biting your lips."
"It makes me uncomfortable when you. . . ."

The nurse often makes observations that can be called to the patient's attention. The patient may be showing signs of anxiety—trembling, clench-

[9] Brown, Martha Montgomery, and Grace R. Fowler: *Psychodynamic Nursing*, 2nd ed. Philadelphia: Saunders, 1961, p. 98.
[10] Schwartz and Shockley, *op. cit.*, p. 236.

ing his fists, biting his nails or lips, smoking endlessly, or other restless mannerisms—of which he is unaware. Or he may have begun to hallucinate actively. He may seem perplexed, fearful, far off in thought, angry, or sad. On the other hand, the nurse herself may have become uncomfortable as the result of certain behavior on the part of the patient. In any of these or similar instances, the nurse can bring her observations to the awareness of the patient and encourage their mutual understanding of the behavior or feeling through discussion. This technique is especially useful in relating to mute patients. By voicing her perceptions, such as, "You seem deep in thought," "Your expression conveys bewilderment to me," or "You appear more comfortable with me today," she offers the patient something to which he may respond when ready. Thus she avoids pressing questions on him, yet does not enter into a mutual state of muteness.

By calling the patient's attention to what is happening to him, the nurse seeks to encourage the patient's noticing for himself so that he can do the describing. Then the nurse and the patient can compare their observations.

9. ENCOURAGING DESCRIPTION OF PERCEPTIONS . . . asking the patient to verbalize what he perceives.

"Tell me when you feel anxious."
"What is happening?"
"What does the voice seem to be saying?"

If the nurse is to understand the patient, she must come to see things as they seem to him. The patient should feel free to describe his perceptions to the nurse. In addition to describing his past experiences, he should be alerted to becoming aware of signs of anxiety, thoughts that interrupt and normally would be pushed aside,[11] hallucinatory phenomena, and other disturbing events, feelings, sensations, or ideas. When possible, these should be described to the nurse as they are occurring. Both the patient and the nurse need such descriptions if they are to come to understand the reasons for the patient's behavior. These descriptions are the raw material from which the understandings will be drawn.[12]

Rogers[13] states,

> It is natural to expect that with increasing security in clinical experience there will be an increasing variety of attempts to communicate the fact that the therapist is endeavoring to achieve the internal frame of reference of the client,

[11] Sullivan, Harry Stack: *Conceptions of Modern Psychiatry*, 2nd ed. New York: Norton, 1953, pp. 200–201.

[12] Peplau, Hildegard E.: "Talking with Patients," *Am. J. Nursing*, **60**:964–67, July 1960.

[13] Rogers, Carl R.: *Client-centered Therapy*. Boston: Houghton Mifflin, 1951, p. 31.

and is trying to see with him as deeply as the client sees, or even more deeply than the latter is able at the moment to perceive.

He[14] adds,

. . . it would appear that for me, as counselor, to focus my whole attention and effort upon understanding and perceiving as the client perceives and understands, is a striking operational demonstration of the belief I have in the worth and significance of this individual client.

Nurses sometimes feel that encouraging the patient to describe his ideas tends to fix more firmly in his mind the irrational and delusional thoughts he may have. Suicidal and aggressive thoughts and feelings are especially anxiety-provoking for the nurse. However, Schwartz and Shockley point out that the patient may not have to act out if he feels free to talk about his difficulties. Talking may make it unnecessary for the patient to behave in a manner harmful to himself or others.[15]

10. ENCOURAGING COMPARISON . . . asking that similarities and differences be noted.

"Was this something like. . . ?"
"Have you had similar experiences?"

Comparing ideas or experiences or interpersonal relationships brings out many recurring themes. Seeing the similarities helps the patient become aware of the continuity in his life, and noting differences helps him to evaluate the influence of each event or person individually. Peplau emphasizes the nurse's "being herself" as another means of assisting the patient to become aware of likenesses and differences among people.[16] Again, it is obvious that relationships are based on more than words alone. The whole person who is the nurse is relating to the patient. Her feelings and behavior communicate more than her words.

While comparisons are to be encouraged, it is rarely helpful for the nurse to introduce experiences from her own life for this purpose. Too frequently the result is a discussion focused on the needs and problems of the nurse.

11. RESTATING . . . repeating the main idea expressed.

Patient. I can't sleep. I stay awake all night.
Nurse. You have difficulty sleeping.

[14] *Ibid.*, p. 35.
[15] Schwartz and Shockley, *op. cit.*, p. 234.
[16] Peplau, *Interpersonal Relations in Nursing*, p. 52.

Patient. The fellow that is my mate died at war and is pending me yet to marry.

Nurse. You were going to marry him, but he died during the war.

What the patient has said is repeated in approximately or nearly the same words that he has used. This restatement gives evidence to the patient that an idea has been communicated effectively. He is encouraged to continue. Or, if his thoughts have been misunderstood, he can reword and restate them until he makes himself clear.

An additional benefit, Wolberg feels, is that, "Recasting certain statements into different words brings out related aspects of the material that may have escaped the patient's attention."[17]

12. REFLECTING . . . directing back to the patient questions, feelings, and ideas.

Patient. Do you think I should tell the doctor. . . ?

Nurse. Do *you* think you should?

Patient. My brother spends all my money and then has the nerve to ask for more.

Nurse. This causes you to feel angry.

Reflection encourages the patient to bring forth and accept as part of himself his own ideas and feelings. When the patient asks what he should think or do or feel, the nurse can ask, "What do *you* think?" or "What are *your* feelings?" The nurse thereby indicates that it is the patient's point of view that has value. Thus she acknowledges his right to have opinions, to make decisions, and to think for himself. As the nurse shows that she expects him to be able to do these things, he too comes to think of himself as a capable person—as a relatively integrated whole rather than the incorporated parts of others. When the patient expresses feelings and ideas, the nurse can recognize and accept them, acknowledge their existence, and reflect them back by noting, "You think . . ." and "You feel. . . ." This helps the patient to accept them as belonging to him. Karnosh and Mereness suggest that the nurse's skillful reflection of the patient's comments makes obvious her interest in hearing as much as the patient needs to tell.[18] Reflection, Brammer and Shostrom[19] state,

> . . . focuses on the subjective element of what the client says. Reflection emphasizes the pronoun "you" in the phrases, "you feel" and "you think."

[17] Wolberg, *op. cit.*, p. 177.

[18] Karnosh, Louis J., and Dorothy Mereness: *Psychiatry for Nurses*, 5th ed. St. Louis: C. V. Mosby Co., 1958, p. 43.

[19] Brammer and Shostrom, *op. cit.*, p. 174.

Reflection serves a useful purpose in that it leads the client to think of the feelings and ideas he is expressing as part of his own personality and not outside himself.

The patient is encouraged to separate himself from the personalities of others and to become a person in his own right.

13. FOCUSING . . . concentrating on a single point.

"This point seems worth looking at more closely."

Focusing on a single idea or even a single word can often be very valuable. In effect the nurse says, "This seems important. It is worth spending some time in understanding it now." It is an especially useful technique when the patient jumps rapidly from one thought to another. If severe anxiety is present, however, and the patient is thereby prevented from focusing, the nurse should not persist. As anxiety lessens, the nurse may again utilize this technique.

14. EXPLORING . . . delving further into a subject or idea.

"Tell me more about that."
"Would you describe it more fully?"
"What kind of work?"

Exploring more fully certain ideas, experiences, or relationships is frequently indicated. Many patients deal only superficially with each topic they bring up, as if testing to see whether the nurse is really interested enough to look further or as if to say that nothing of importance has ever happened in their lives. Wolberg suggests that once a theme or trend is identified, it should be explored in as elaborate detail as possible.[20] While the nurse should recognize when to delve further, she should refrain from probing or prying. If the patient chooses not to elaborate, the nurse should respect the patient's wishes.

15. GIVING INFORMATION . . . making available the facts the patient needs.

"My name is. . . ."
"Visiting hours are. . . ."
"My purpose in being here is. . . ."
"I'm taking you to the. . . ."

[20] Wolberg, *op. cit.*, p. 411.

Informing the patient of the facts when he asks questions—or in other ways indicates the need for information—builds up trust as well as gives the patient a greater body of knowledge from which to make decisions or come to realistic conclusions. Peplau states that a nurse, functioning in the role of resource person, may give specific, needed information that will assist the patient to understand his problem and the situation.[21] If the nurse is not acquainted with the body of knowledge in question, she can truthfully state that she does not know. Then she can endeavor to find out or to refer the patient to someone who has the answers. Areas of information not to be neglected are the role of the nurse and the purpose of the nurse-patient relationship. The nurse should inform the patient of the amount of time she will spend with him, how frequently she will talk with him, and the length or duration of the relationship if this has been predetermined. If she will be recording the interaction, the patient should be told the purpose of the notes. A distinction should be made between this therapeutic relationship and other social relationships the patient may be establishing. In all these things the nurse will usually find that she can be quite direct, avoiding vague and misleading statements.

16. SEEKING CLARIFICATION . . . seeking to make clear that which is not meaningful or that which is vague.

"I'm not sure that I follow."
"What would you say is the main point of what you said?"

Clarification should be sought at each step of the way. The patient is usually quite aware when he is not being understood. Eventually he may cease trying to communicate. Peplau[22] states that it

> . . . is always possible to ask: What did you have in mind? Have I heard you correctly? Have I understood what you mean, let me repeat what you said? Perhaps you can help me to get clear on what you mean? Perhaps both of us are looking at this issue or problem from a different standpoint; maybe we'd better talk about its meaning to each.

Fromm-Reichmann notes that it is not necessary to understand everything the patient says as long as the nurse is frank about it and does not make pretenses.[23] Not only is the nurse benefited by clarification, Sullivan points out, but attempts to discover what the patient is talking about can lead to his becoming more clear himself on what he means. The patient's grasp on life is thus to some extent enhanced.[24]

[21] Peplau, *Interpersonal Relations in Nursing*, p. 21.
[22] *Ibid.*, pp. 293–94.
[23] Fromm-Reichmann, Frieda: *Principles of Intensive Psychotherapy*. Chicago: University of Chicago Press, 1950, p. 18.
[24] Sullivan, Harry Stack: *The Psychiatric Interview*. New York: Norton, 1954, pp. 23–24.

17. PRESENTING REALITY . . . offering for consideration that which is real.

"I see no one else in the room."
"That sound was a car backfiring."
"Your mother is not here; I'm a nurse."

When it is obvious that the patient is misinterpreting reality, the nurse can indicate that which is real. She does this not by way of arguing with the patient or belittling his own experiences, but rather by calmly and quietly expressing her own perceptions or the facts in the situation. The intent here is merely to indicate an alternate line of thought for the patient to consider, not to "convince" the patient that he is in error.

18. VOICING DOUBT . . . expressing uncertainty as to the reality of the patient's perceptions.

"Isn't that unusual?"
"Really?"
"That's hard to believe."

Another means of responding to distortions of reality is to express doubt. Such expression permits the patient to become aware that others do not necessarily perceive events in the same way or draw the same conclusions that he does. This does not mean that he will alter his point of view, but at least he will be encouraged to reconsider and to re-evaluate what has occurred. And the nurse has neither agreed nor disagreed, yet, at the same time, she has not let misinterpretations and distortions of reality pass uncommented upon. Sullivan[25] expresses this quite well when he states,

> . . . you should first confirm, by asking the most natural questions that would follow, that the patient intended to say what he did. . . . Having made sure that the patient's statement was as bad as it sounded—that he is entertaining an idea which is not only wrong, but also, in a sense, does violence to the possibility of his living in a social situation among others—you do not then say, "Oh, yes, yes. How interesting!" You rather say, "I can scarcely believe it. What on earth gives you that impression?" You note a marked exception. . . . at least you note your exception and do not agree tacitly.

19. SEEKING CONSENSUAL VALIDATION . . . searching for mutual understanding, for accord in the meaning of words.

"Tell me whether my understanding of it agrees with yours."
"Are you using this word to convey the idea. . . ?"

[25] Sullivan, *The Psychiatric Interview*, p. 235.

For verbal communication to be meaningful, it is imperative that the words conveying the ideas and concepts being discussed have essentially the same meaning for all participants. The nurse may have to suggest, "Are you using this phrase to convey the idea . . . ?" or "Perhaps my understanding of this word differs from yours." Otherwise, nurse and patient may find that each is using the same words differently and that no communication is taking place. Sullivan suggests that the therapist listen with critical interest, asking himself whether what he hears could have any other meaning than that which first occurs to him, asking questions when indicated to be sure that he knows what he is being told. As the patient makes himself clearer to the listener, he becomes more clear in his own mind as to what he means.[26] Peplau adds that both nurse and patient have preconceptions about the meanings of words, but that a common reference for the word can usually be arrived at through observation and discussion.[27] To facilitate such consensual validation, the nurse should make every effort to avoid expressions that can easily be misinterpreted or misunderstood.

20. VERBALIZING THE IMPLIED . . . voicing what the patient has hinted at or suggested.

Patient. I can't talk to you or to anyone. It's a waste of time.
Nurse. Is it your feeling that no one understands?

Patient. My wife pushes me around just like my mother and sister did.
Nurse. Is it your impression that women are domineering?

To put into words what has been implied or said only indirectly tends to make the discussion less obscure. The nurse should be as direct as she can be, without being obtuse or unfeelingly blunt. The patient himself may find it difficult to be direct—to find the appropriate words or the courage to say them—or he may be testing the nurse to see whether she is really striving to grasp what he says. The nurse should take care to express only what is fairly obvious; otherwise she gets into the realm of offering interpretations. In Sullivan's words, ". . . putting the obvious into words often markedly improves things."[28] Verbalizing the implied goes one step beyond restatement in that it clarifies that which is implicit, rather than explicit, in that which has just been said. It reflects relationships or meanings for the patient that have been suggested or implied in the thoughts or feelings brought out by the patient's responses.[29]

[26] *Ibid.*, pp. 20–21.
[27] Peplau, *Interpersonal Relations in Nursing*, p. 291.
[28] Sullivan, *The Psychiatric Interview*, p. 230.
[29] Brammer and Shostrom, *op. cit.*, p. 247.

21. ENCOURAGING EVALUATION . . . asking the patient to appraise the quality of his experiences.

"What are your feelings in regard to. . . ?"
"Does this contribute to your discomfort?"

The patient is asked to consider people and events in the light of his own set of values and to evaluate the way in which they affect him personally. He is thereby discouraged from adopting without appraisal the opinions and values of others, including those of the nurse. Rogers notes that some patients make great efforts to have the therapist exercise the valuing function but stresses that it is the therapist's task to consistently keep "the locus of evaluation" with the patient.[30]

22. ATTEMPTING TO TRANSLATE INTO FEELINGS . . . seeking to verbalize the feelings that are being expressed only indirectly.

Patient. I'm dead.
Nurse. Are you suggesting that you feel lifeless?
or Is it that life seems without meaning?

Patient. I'm way out in the ocean.
Nurse. It must be lonely.
or You seem to feel deserted.

Often what the patient says, when taken literally, seems meaningless or far removed from reality. To understand, the nurse must concentrate on what the patient might be feeling in order to express himself as he does.[31] Peplau suggests that the nurse ask herself what the patient is saying that he cannot say in any other way. She then must desymbolize what is actually said to find clues to the underlying meaning.[32] Wolberg aptly speaks of this process as "reaching" for feelings that lie behind verbalization.[33] Only then can the nurse attempt to verbalize the feelings that the patient has difficulty putting into words. For example, the patient who sees the personnel as "giants" is likely to feel insignificant and powerless by comparison. For the nurse to introduce these feelings into the discussion is likely to have more value than for her to discuss the "giants" as such. It is the latent meaning of the expression rather than the actual content that

[30] Rogers, *Client-centered Therapy*, p. 150.
[31] Hays, Joyce Samhammer: "Focusing on Feelings," *Nursing Outlook,* **10**:332 33, May 1962.
[32] Peplau, *Interpersonal Relations in Nursing*, p. 295.
[33] Wolberg, *op. cit.*, p. 166.

demands the nurse's attention.[34] Rogers points out that responding primarily in terms of the feelings expressed—rather than the content—gives the patient the satisfaction of feeling deeply understood and enables him to express further feelings.[35]

23. SUGGESTING COLLABORATION . . . offering to share, to strive, to work together with the patient for his benefit.

"Perhaps you and I can discuss and discover what produces your anxiety."

The nurse seeks to offer the patient a relationship in which he can identify his problems in living with others, grow emotionally, and improve his ability to form satisfying relationships with others. She offers to do things not *for* him or *to* him, but *with* him. Peplau speaks of a cooperative relationship in which both the nurse and the patient can become aware of the nature of the problems or tasks and how they can be met.[36] "To encourage the patient to participate in identifying and assessing his problem is to engage him as an active partner in an enterprise of great concern to him."[37] Sullivan states that he always tries to outline for the patient what he sees as a major difficulty in his living with others with the implication that if they "work together," he has hopes that they will get somewhere with the problem.[38]

24. SUMMARIZING . . . organizing and summing up that which has gone before.

"Have I got this straight?"
"You've said that. . . ."
"During the past hour you and I have discussed. . . ."

Summarization seeks to bring together the important points of the discussion and to give each participant an awareness of the progress made toward greater understanding. It omits the irrelevant and organizes the pertinent aspects of the interaction. It allows both nurse and patient to

[34] Brown and Fowler, *op. cit.*, p. 98.
[35] Rogers, Carl R.: *Counseling and Psychotherapy*. Boston: Houghton Mifflin, 1942, p. 141.
[36] Peplau, *Interpersonal Relations in Nursing*, p. 50.
[37] *Ibid.*, p. 23.
[38] Sullivan, *The Psychiatric Interview*, p. 92.

depart with the same ideas in mind and provides a sense of closure at the completion of each discussion. This summing up can be done periodically throughout the discussion or only at its close. But no matter who does it or how frequently it occurs, summarization is a valuable part of each exchange. For it is during periods of summarization that the nurse and the patient strive to grasp the significance of what has been said, to formulate the meaning of the data, and to achieve new understandings. Wolberg mentions that for the patient who rambles and becomes so engrossed in detail that he loses sight of the interrelationship of the topics he's presenting, summarization is helpful. It pulls together what seems to be disorganized material.[39] Brammer and Shostrom suggest three alternatives. The therapist himself can review the content and essential feelings expressed during the interview. The patient can be asked to relate what he feels he has accomplished or what the situation appears to be now. Or the therapist and the patient can look together at what has been achieved.[40] Perhaps in the nursing relationship the summary can be less formal, but this does not mean that it should be omitted. A simple, "Have you and I learned anything from today's conversation?" may be quite sufficient.

25. ENCOURAGING FORMULATION OF A PLAN OF ACTION . . . asking the patient to consider kinds of behavior likely to be appropriate in future situations.

> "What could you do to let your anger out harmlessly?"
> "Next time this comes up, what might you do to handle it?"

It may be helpful for the patient to plan for the future what he might do to handle various interpersonal situations that he finds disturbing, such as those in which he is provoked to anger or in which he is hesitant or shy or anxious. Talking over each situation in an attempt to better understand it will, of course, precede this "plan of action." And whatever plans are made should be the patient's, not the nurse's. While it should be recognized that preplanning in itself will not solve the problem, there is the likelihood that later behavior will be guided by such thinking rather than by impulse alone. In addition, the nurse may encourage the patient to role-play or act out with her such situations in advance, as another means of preparation. In a broad sense, the entire nurse-patient relationship is an experience of this sort—a preview of future relationships of a more reciprocal nature in which the patient may find—and give—acceptance, respect, and understanding.

[39] Wolberg, *op. cit.*, pp. 176–77.
[40] Brammer and Shostrom, *op. cit.*, p. 202.

INTERPERSONAL TECHNIQUES

THERAPEUTIC TECHNIQUES	EXAMPLES
1. *Using Silence*	
2. *Accepting*	Yes. Uh hmm. I follow what you said. Nodding.
3. *Giving Recognition*	Good morning Mr. S. You've tooled a leather wallet. I notice that you've combed your hair.
4. *Offering Self*	I'll sit with you awhile. I'll stay here with you. I'm interested in your comfort.
5. *Giving Broad Openings*	Is there something you'd like to talk about? What are you thinking about? Where would you like to begin?
6. *Offering General Leads*	Go on. And then? Tell me about it.
7. *Placing the Event in Time or in Sequence*	What seemed to lead up to. . . ? Was this before or after. . . ? When did this happen?
8. *Making Observations*	You appear tense. Are you uncomfortable when you. . . ? I notice that you're biting your lips. It makes me uncomfortable when you. . . .
9. *Encouraging Description of Perceptions*	Tell me when you feel anxious. What is happening? What does the voice seem to be saying?
10. *Encouraging Comparison*	Was this something like. . . ? Have you had similar experiences?
11. *Restating*	**Patient.** I can't sleep. I stay awake all night. **Nurse.** You have difficulty sleeping. **Patient.** The fellow that is my mate died at war and is pending me yet to marry. **Nurse.** You were going to marry him, but he died during the war.

THERAPEUTIC TECHNIQUES	EXAMPLES
12. *Reflecting*	**Patient.** Do you think I should tell t doctor. . . ? **Nurse.** Do *you* think you should? **Patient.** My brother spends all n money and then has the nerve to a for more. **Nurse.** This causes you to feel angry.
13. *Focusing*	This point seems worth looking at mo closely.
14. *Exploring*	Tell me more about that. Would you describe it more fully? What kind of work?
15. *Giving Information*	My name is. . . . Visiting hours are. . . . My purpose in being here is. . . . I'm taking you to the. . . .
16. *Seeking Clarification*	I'm not sure that I follow. What would you say is the main poi of what you said?
17. *Presenting Reality*	I see no one else in the room. That sound was a car backfiring. Your mother is not here; I'm a nurse.
18. *Voicing Doubt*	Isn't that unusual? Really? That's hard to believe.
19. *Seeking Consensual Validation*	Tell me whether my understanding of agrees with yours. Are you using this word to convey th idea. . . ?
20. *Verbalizing the Implied*	**Patient.** I can't talk to you or to anyon It's a waste of time. **Nurse.** Is it your feeling that no o understands? **Patient.** My wife pushes me around ju like my mother and sister did. **Nurse.** Is it your impression that wom are domineering?
21. *Encouraging Evaluation*	What are your feelings in regard to. . . Does this contribute to your discon fort?

THERAPEUTIC TECHNIQUES	EXAMPLES
2. *Attempting to Translate into Feelings*	**Patient.** I'm dead. **Nurse.** Are you suggesting that you feel lifeless? **or** Is it that life seems without meaning? **Patient.** I'm way out in the ocean. **Nurse.** It must be lonely. **or** You seem to feel deserted.
3. *Suggesting Collaboration*	Perhaps you and I can discuss and discover what produces your anxiety.
4. *Summarizing*	Have I got this straight? You've said that. . . . During the past hour you and I have discussed. . . .
5. *Encouraging Formulation of a Plan of Action*	What could you do to let your anger out harmlessly? Next time this comes up, what might you do to handle it?

Nontherapeutic Techniques

1. REASSURING . . . indicating that there is no cause for anxiety.

"I wouldn't worry about. . . ."
"Everything will be all right."
"You're coming along fine."

To attempt to dispel the patient's anxiety by implying that there is not sufficient reason for it to exist is to completely devaluate the patient's own feelings. Hence, no value is placed on the patient's judgment. The nurse communicates only her lack of understanding and empathy. If it is the patient's progress she wants to comment upon, she can offer concrete examples of changes that have occurred rather than state, "You're doing fine" or other equally vague reassurances that have little or no meaning. Burton tells us that giving reassurance is a common error. It makes the person giving it feel better for a short time but is meaningless to the patient. She adds,[1]

In the first place, the person giving the reassurance is not sure that someone will feel better, or will live, or will have a satisfying outcome from an operation. It is hoped that he will, but that is all. Furthermore, the reassurance is belittling to the person who has the problem or worry. . . . An immediate effect of this response is to block the person from expressing further feeling. In the person who is blocked by someone's reassurance there is a negative feeling stirred up which says, "There's no point in trying to tell her anything because she won't understand; she will ridicule my fear, making me feel foolish."

Sullivan concurs by stating that such verbalisms—the attempt to do magic with language—reassures the therapist rather than the patient.[2] Magic, he

[1] Burton, Genevieve: *Personal, Impersonal, and Interpersonal Relations.* New York: Springer, 1958, p. 178.

[2] Sullivan, Harry Stack: *The Psychiatric Interview.* New York: Norton, 1954, pp. 217–18.

says, cannot be done with reassuring words. The real magic is done by the patient, not the therapist, and occurs in the interpersonal relationship. There is absolutely no justification for trying to reassure, unless you are able to document what you say. "All in all, when you can't reassure a person except by magic, the sensible thing is not to try."[3]

2. GIVING APPROVAL . . . sanctioning the patient's ideas or behavior.

"That's good."
"I'm glad that you. . . ."

To state that what the patient is doing, feeling, or saying is "good" is to imply that its opposite is "bad." Approval, then, tends to limit the patient's freedom to think, speak, or act in a way that displeases the nurse. It also leads the patient to strive for praise rather than progress. Peplau states that praise arouses undue ambition, competitiveness, and a sense of superiority. The possibilities for learning are closed off, as the patient speaks and acts in terms of what brings approval. Eventually the patient comes to focus almost exclusively on what will bring approval. She adds, "Praise and blame, good and bad, right and wrong, leave nurses only a two-sided coin with which to operate in their relations with patients. Focusing on the steps in learning allows infinite variety in relations with patients. . . ."[4] While approval and disapproval are likely to alter undesirable behavior, Burton notes that such changes, though they come about quickly, are not usually lasting. For as soon as the motivating force is removed, the original behavior returns.[5] Hence, no learning has occurred.

3. REJECTING . . . refusing to consider or showing contempt for the patient's ideas or behavior.

"Let's not discuss. . . ."
"I don't want to hear about. . . ."

When any topic is rejected, it is closed off from exploration. When the patient himself is rejected, therapeutic interaction ceases. Fromm-Reichmann points out that the insecure therapist is likely to be afraid of the patient's anxiety-producing experiences. He thwarts the patient's expressions by giving premature reassurances that he needs himself. Consequently, certain areas of the patient's experience are not submitted to investigation.[6]

[3] *Ibid.*, pp. 227–29.
[4] Peplau, Hildegard E.: *Interpersonal Relations in Nursing.* New York: G. P. Putnam's Sons, 1952, pp. 235–37.
[5] Burton, *op. cit.*, p. 160.
[6] Fromm-Reichmann, Frieda: *Principles of Intensive Psychotherapy.* Chicago: University of Chicago Press, 1950, pp. 24–25.

According to Burton, the patient tends to feel rejected by the nurse when she is fearful of permitting him to express his feelings and to reveal his problems. He then may avoid help rather than risk further rejection.[7] It is important for the nurse to know herself—to identify kinds of behavior or ideas that make her anxious—and to seek help for her problems. Otherwise, she is likely to add new problems to those with which the patient is already struggling.

4. DISAPPROVING . . . denouncing the patient's behavior or ideas.

"That's bad."
"I'd rather you wouldn't. . . ."

Disapproval implies that the nurse has the right to pass judgment on the patient's thoughts and actions. It further implies that the patient is expected to please the nurse. Schwartz and Shockley suggest that the nurse accept the patient for what he is, being neither moralistic nor conditional in this acceptance.[8] They add,[9]

> It is important for a number of reasons to find an alternative to the moralistic attitude in relating with patients. The patient may have been criticized, condemned, and rejected in the past, and these attitudes have contributed to his illness. A blaming and punishing attitude may reinforce his loneliness and hopelessness by confirming his feeling that people cannot or will not understand him. These moralistic attitudes might take the nurse's attention away from the patient's needs and from her relations with him and direct it toward her own feelings.

It is important for the nurse to acknowledge that the patient has a right to behave as he does, for a patient's sick behavior is no more right or wrong, good or bad, than is the pain of a somatic illness.[10] Brammer and Shostrom add that approval and disapproval tend to "have the unfortunate effect of rigidifying the client's thinking."[11] At times the patient's behavior may be so extreme as to cause harm or discomfort to others. Rather than insist, "You're behaving badly" or "That's wrong," she might say, "You are hurting Mr. S., we cannot allow you to do this," or "We will have to move you from the dayroom for now, you're making Mr. S. very uncomfortable by speaking to him this way." Thus the nurse informs the patient of the effects of his actions instead of offering value judgments.

[7] Burton, *op. cit.*, pp. 195–96.

[8] Schwartz, Morris S., and Emmy Lanning Shockley: *The Nurse and the Mental Patient.* New York: Russell Sage Foundation, 1956, p. 255.

[9] *Ibid.*, p. 269.

[10] Matheney, Ruth V., and Mary Topalis: *Psychiatric Nursing,* 3rd ed. St. Louis: C. V. Mosby Co., 1961, p. 80.

[11] Brammer, Lawrence M., and Everett L. Shostrom: *Therapeutic Psychology: Fundamentals of Counseling and Psychotherapy.* Englewood Cliffs, N.J.: Prentice-Hall, 1960, p. 197.

5. AGREEING . . . indicating accord with the patient.

"That's right."
"I agree."

While approval indicates that the patient is "good" rather than "bad," agreeing indicates that he is "right" rather than "wrong." Furthermore, agreement gives the patient the impression that he is "right" because his opinion is the same as that of the nurse. Opinions and conclusions should be exclusively the patient's, not shared with the nurse. When the nurse agrees with the patient, she leaves him with little opportunity to modify his point of view subsequently. Actual agreement tends to make the patient feel that he cannot later change his position without admitting error.[12] Rather than take sides for or against the patient, the nurse can better use her time to help the patient gather the data needed to form his own opinions and draw conclusions. If she is aware of information the patient needs, she can make this available to him. But to evaluate the data is a task for the patient. This does not mean that she cannot say, "That's right," when the patient asks, "This is Thursday, isn't it?" This is the acknowledgment of a fact. At no time, however, should the nurse agree with delusional ideas.

Since accord is involved in both, it is important to distinguish between agreement and consensual validation. To agree is to indicate accord with the patient's system of values—with his opinions, conclusions, or point of view. Consensual validation refers to shared understanding of the meaning of words. No value judgment is involved. It is not a question of whether a word or an expression is right or wrong but whether it conveys similar meaning to both nurse and patient. Without consensual validation no communication can occur. Shared opinions and judgments are not necessary to effective communication.

6. DISAGREEING . . . opposing the patient's ideas.

"That's wrong."
"I definitely disagree with. . . ."
"I don't believe that."

Conversely, to disagree is to imply that the patient is "wrong." Disagreement places the nurse in opposition to the patient. Consequently, he feels called on to defend himself. To defend one's ideas tends to strengthen them. If these are delusional ideas, the nurse may be building up what she had intended to tear down. Rogers feels that when the therapist thinks in evaluative terms, i.e., becomes judgmental, he is seeing the patient as an object rather than as a person, and to that extent respects the patient less.[13]

[12] *Ibid.*, p. 197.
[13] Rogers, Carl R.: *Client-centered Therapy*. Boston: Houghton Mifflin, 1951, p. 45.

Acceptance of the patient as he is frees him to perceive new meanings and new goals. Rogers[14] states:

> . . . only as the therapist is completely willing that *any* outcome, *any* direction, may be chosen—only then does he realize the vital strength of the capacity and potentiality of the individual for constructive action. It is as he is willing for death to be the choice, that life is chosen; for neuroticism to be the choice that a healthy normality is chosen.

These are strong words—anxiety-provoking perhaps. But while disagreement confines the patient, acceptance frees him to grow emotionally. The nurse cannot grow for the patient. She can only provide a relationship in which growth is possible—not mandatory.

7. ADVISING . . . telling the patient what to do.

"I think you should. . . ."
"Why don't you. . . ?"

When the nurse tells the patient what he should think or how he should behave, she implies that she knows what is best for him and that he is incapable of any self-direction. Peplau states that advice acts to prevent the patient from struggling with and thinking through his problems.[15] Moreover, it is most likely that the patient has already received innumerable suggestions and advice from his family and friends. "If the matter were simply one of telling patients what is wrong with their feelings . . . most—if not all—of the psychiatric patients in psychiatric institutions would probably be well. . . ."[16] There is a difference between giving advice and giving information. By giving advice, the nurse takes away from the patient the responsibility that is rightly his.[17] To give advice is to keep patients in a state "of immature dependence upon the judgment and guidance of others. . . ."[18] To give information, on the other hand, is to supply the patient with additional data from which he can later formulate his own course of action.

8. PROBING . . . persistent questioning of the patient.

"Now tell me about. . . ."
"Tell me your life history."

Probing tends to make the patient feel used. He feels valued only for what he can give. It places him on the defensive. He may respond with anger,

[14] *Ibid.*, pp. 48–49.
[15] Peplau, *op cit.*, p. 48.
[16] *Ibid.*, p. 251.
[17] Burton, *op. cit.*, pp. 180–81.
[18] Fromm-Reichmann, *op. cit.*, p. 208.

with distortions or evasions, or cease to respond entirely. As Burton aptly notes, "Probing belongs in surgery, not in counseling."[19] Arieti[20] states,

Each question is experienced by the schizophrenic as an imposition, or an intrusion into his private life, and will increase his anxiety, his hostility, and his desire to desocialize. The request for information is not seldom interpreted by the patient as "an attempt to take away something from him."

While the response of the schizophrenic patient may be extreme, it is not unusual for any person to resent this technique, particularly the patient under the stress of illness. Often the nurse is not aware that she has been persistently questioning the patient until she looks over the notes she has taken during the interaction. Especially when the patient is quiet or withdrawn and answers only briefly or not at all, the nurse tends to become increasingly anxious and increasingly persistent in her questioning, without being aware of what is happening. If the nurse can focus on the patient and his discomfort and can "put herself in his place" during the discussion, she is likely to find herself less anxious and more likely to be "in tune with" the patient.

9. CHALLENGING . . . demanding proof from the patient.

"But how can you be President of the United States?"
"If you're dead, why is your heart beating?"

Often the nurse feels that if she can challenge the patient to prove his unrealistic ideas and/or perceptions, he will realize that he has no "proof" and will be forced to acknowledge what is "true." She forgets that delusional ideas serve a purpose for the patient and are not given up so readily. Moreover, these ideas conceal feelings and meet needs that are real. When challenged, the patient tends only to strengthen and expand his misinterpretations of reality, as he seeks support for his point of view. Only as the nurse is able to discover the unmet needs and help the patient meet them in reality is there likely to be less need for the unrealistic ideas and perceptions.

10. TESTING . . . appraising the patient's degree of insight.

"What day is this?"
"Do you know what kind of a hospital this is?"
"Do you still have the idea that. . . ?"

It is not uncommon for the nurse to feel that she must convince the patient of the extent of his incapacity and have him agree that this is so.

[19] Burton, *op. cit.*, p. 184.
[20] Arieti, Silvano: "Schizophrenia: Other Aspects; Psychotherapy," *American Handbook of Psychiatry*, New York: Basic Books, 1959, p. 499.

Actually the nurse is saying, "Admit that you are sick and need help." Paradoxically, she demands that the patient have insight into his very lack of insight. For him to agree that this is so—at her insistence—meets only the nurse's needs, not those of the patient. It is preferable to assume the best about the patient, e.g., the nurse saying, "Tell me about what took place," rather than asking, "Can you remember what happened?" The latter implies that the patient is probably not capable of recall. As Sullivan has noted, "There is no reason to pronounce the patient insane as a preliminary to helping him to regain his sanity."[21]

11. DEFENDING . . . attempting to protect someone or something from verbal attack.

"This hospital has a fine reputation."
"No one here would lie to you."
"But Dr. B. is a very able psychiatrist."
"I'm sure that he has your welfare in mind when he. . . ."

To defend what the patient has criticized is to imply that he has no right to express his impressions, opinions, or feelings. Telling the patient that his criticism is unjust or unfounded does not change his feelings. The feelings still exist and are in need of expression. But when the nurse becomes defensive, she causes the patient to feel that he should discontinue such expression. As a result, the patient often feels only more strongly that his impressions are valid—that he has uncovered a weakness that others are trying to conceal. Burton[22] states that the nurse

> . . . accepts the patient's right to feel as he does, without necessarily agreeing with him. . . . When we fly to the defense of someone we are implying that the other person needs to be defended. Whereas if we really have faith in the person or profession criticized we should not feel that defense is necessary. Furthermore, when we defend someone we are usually lining ourselves up with that person against the person making the criticism.

Perhaps the most difficult criticisms to accept are those directed at the nurse herself. But if she feels relatively secure as a person, she will find that genuine acceptance and understanding of the patient make defending herself unnecessary.

12. REQUESTING AN EXPLANATION . . . asking the patient to provide the reasons for thoughts, feelings, behavior, and events.

"Why do you think that?"
"Why do you feel this way?"
"Why did you do that?"

[21] Sullivan, *op. cit.*, p. 65.
[22] Burton, *op. cit.*, p. 184.

There is a difference between asking the patient to *describe* what is occurring or has taken place and asking him to explain *why*. The former is to be encouraged. When an explanation is sought, however, it is often necessary for the patient to make up for his lack of sufficient understanding by inventing a reason, giving partial answers, or expanding his delusional system to provide the requested explanations. It is only after much learning has taken place that the patient is ready to attempt to explain what has happened. Peplau notes that the nurse often automatically asks, "Why?" or "Why not?" She adds,[23]

> More often than not a "why" question has an intimidating effect. It has a ring of familiarity and is frequently reminiscent of earlier experiences when mother or teacher reiterated "Why don't you do this" or "Why can't you tell me" or some similarly coercing "why" question. Moreover, if the patient knew why he wasn't sleeping or hungry or comfortable, he would most probably deal with the situation. A "why" question asks for reasons which the patient is not likely to know immediately. He can discover them with help. But, in order to discover them, the patient requires some raw data—he must recall, for example, what actually went on. . . . The reasons can be generalized from these data; then the "why" question can be answered.

13. INDICATING THE EXISTENCE OF AN EXTERNAL SOURCE . . . attributing the source of thoughts, feelings, and behavior to others or to outside influences.

"What makes you say that?"
"Who told you that you were Jesus?"
"What made you do that?"

The nurse can ask, "What happened?" or "What events led you to draw such a conclusion?" But to question "What made you think that?" seems to imply that the patient was made or compelled to think in a certain way—that someone or something was the cause for the patient's ideas, feelings, or actions. Usually the nurse does not intend to suggest that the source is external. She really thinks that she is asking the patient to describe the way in which something came about. But its probable meaning to the patient is what must be considered. As Sullivan comments, ". . . you don't know what people mean, or what your words mean to them, until you find out!"[24] Hence, the nurse should always strive to word her comments so as to avoid, insofar as possible, ambiguity. To actually suggest the reality of an external source is to encourage the patient to greater utilization of projection as a means of alleviating anxiety. Moreover, it relieves the patient of responsibility for his own thoughts and actions.

[23] Peplau, Hilldegard E.: "Talking with Patients," *Am. J. Nursing,* **60**:964–67, July 1960.
[24] Sullivan, *op. cit.,* p. 168.

14. BELITTLING FEELINGS EXPRESSED . . . misjudging the degree of the patient's discomfort.

Patient. I have nothing to live for . . . I wish I was dead.
Nurse. Everybody gets down in the dumps.
or I've felt that way sometimes.

When the nurse tries to equate the intense and overwhelming feelings expressed by the patient with those of "everybody" or herself, she implies that the discomfort is temporary, mild, and self-limiting. She then often tells the patient to smile, "buck up," or think of something else. In this way she indicates her lack of empathy and understanding and can offer no constructive assistance. Sullivan warns that anything that causes a patient to feel "small" or insignificant is apt to leave a long-lasting wound. Therefore, the therapist should try very carefully not to belittle or humiliate.[25] As Burton states,[26]

> When you are worried about your own problem, whether big or little, it does not comfort you to know that others are, or have been, in the same boat. . . . when you are concerned with and focusing on your own misery you are not capable of concern about the misery of others.

Of much greater value would be comments such as, "You must be very uncomfortable" or "Would you like to talk about it?" Again, it is important for the nurse to perceive what is taking place from the patient's point of view, not from her own.

15. MAKING STEREOTYPED COMMENTS . . . offering meaningless clichés, trite expressions.

"Nice weather we're having."
"I'm fine, and how are you?"
"It's for your own good."
"Keep your chin up."
"Just listen to your doctor and take part in activities—you'll be home in no time."

It is not unusual for conversations to contain a large proportion of trite expressions, empty words, meaningless clichés, and patterned replies. Such comments lack value in the nurse-patient relationship, just as they do elsewhere. Sullivan asks the therapist to avoid "all impractical meaningless comment. . . ."[27] For the nurse to make empty conversation is to encourage a like response from the patient. And as Sullivan notes, "The more conventional a person's statements are, of course, the more doubtful it is that

[25] *Ibid.*, p. 234.
[26] Burton, *op. cit.*, p. 180.
[27] Sullivan, *op. cit.*, p. 243.

you have any idea of what he really means."[28] Consequently, many words of meaninglessness are exchanged, but nothing is really communicated. If the nurse has nothing meaningful to say, she should say nothing.

Schwartz and Shockley state that the nurse tends to become accustomed to the patient's behavior and adjusts to it by developing a few automatic approaches to him. These responses are of little value.[29] They add,[30]

> Stereotyped responses are also indicated by the way a nurse talks to a patient. When a patient asks the nurse why he should do something which she asks of him the nurse may reply: "It's good for you." "The doctor ordered it." "It will get you well." "Because I want you to do it." None of these responses is necessarily stereotyped, but if her answer is given in a mechanical way as a substitute for a more reasonable and considered explanation, the response may easily become stereotyped. Behind the nurse's automatic responses to a patient may be equally stereotyped attitudes.

16. GIVING LITERAL RESPONSES . . . responding to a figurative comment as though it were a statement of fact.

Patient. I'm an Easter egg.
Nurse. What shade?
or You don't look like one.

Patient. They're looking in my head with television.
Nurse. Try not to watch television.
or With what channel?

Often the patient is at a loss to describe his feelings. When, for example, it seems as though his every thought is known to others, he may say, "They're looking in my head all the time with television." To say that he is an Easter egg may mean that he feels closed away in a shell or conspicuous or less than human. He says these things because at this time it is the best way he has of putting into words the way it seems or feels to him. The feelings he is having are so strange—so foreign to him—that conventional expressions seem highly unsuitable.[31] For the nurse to respond in kind is to indicate her inability to understand when anxiety-producing feelings are being described. Sullivan makes an apt remark: ". . . the patient may get the idea that the psychiatrist is a fool, poorly trained, or part of a plot—no one of which ideas is particularly helpful to therapeutic progress."[32] This is not to imply that all delusional ideas are wholly without

[28] *Ibid.*, p. 21.
[29] Schwartz and Shockley, *op. cit.*, p. 273.
[30] *Ibid.*, p. 274.
[31] Hays, Joyce Samhammer: "Focusing on Feelings," *Nursing Outlook*, **10**:332–33, May 1962.
[32] Sullivan, *op. cit.*, p. 235.

literal meaning to the patient. Perhaps originally this may have been so, but now he undoubtedly takes them literally too. Even so, there is no reason for the nurse to acquire a similar manner of thinking.

17. USING DENIAL . . . refusing to admit that a problem exists.

Patient. I'm nothing.
Nurse. Of course you're something. Everybody is somebody.

Patient. I'm dead.
Nurse. Don't be silly.

We are familiar with the patient who denies that he is sick or has problems of any kind. The nurse, by her comment, tone of voice, or facial expression, often unwittingly uses the same defense to avoid discussion of a problem that she thinks should not exist or an idea that she considers meaningless or perhaps even frightening. In effect, she has closed both her eyes and her mind to the patient's problem. When the nurse uses denial, she shuts off an avenue of discussion and avoids helping the patient to identify and explore his difficulties. Peplau points out that when the nurse "denies the validity of the patient's feelings . . . in order to feel safe the patient may have to give up attending to what he feels and indicate verbal acceptance of what the nurse has indicated he *should* feel."[33]

18. INTERPRETING . . . seeking to make conscious that which is unconscious, telling the patient the meaning of his experience.

"What you really mean is. . . ."
"Unconsciously you're saying. . . ."

Fromm-Reichmann states that to interpret is to "translate the manifestations of that which is barred from awareness into the language of consciousness."[34] The nurse, Peplau tells us, respects the patient's right to have his own feelings and to express them to those who may understand them, but she will not necessarily confront him with the intention of these feelings. While the psychiatrist may interpret directly to the patient, the nurse endangers her usefulness in her other roles—of resource person, mother surrogate—by doing so.[35] She notes that only the psychotherapist is prepared to try to aid in the "release and formulation into awareness of dissociated perceptions, i.e., with unconscious materials."[36] Rogers points out that interpretation seems to indicate a limited confidence in the patient's

[33] Peplau, *op. cit.*, p. 29.
[34] Fromm-Reichmann, Frieda: "Notes on the Development of Treatment of Schizophrenics by Psychoanalytical Psychiatry," *Psychiatry*, 2:263–73, 1948.
[35] Peplau, *op. cit.*, p. 111.
[36] Peplau, Hildegard E.: "Therapeutic Concepts," *Aspects of Psychiatric Nursing*. Section B. League Exchange, No. 26, National League for Nursing, 1957, p. 17.

capacity to cope with his problems.[37] Matheney and Topalis feel that the goal of therapy is helping the patient to develop sufficient emotional maturity so that he can develop and utilize an understanding of his behavior, but they note that such understanding does not come from without.[38] Rogers concurs: ". . . insight is an experience which is achieved, not an experience which can be imposed."[39] Brammer and Shostrom sum up this point of view by noting that a cardinal goal of all therapists for patients is "assisting them toward *self-interpretation,*" since it is the patient who must get the insight, not the therapist.[40] Several drawbacks seem obvious: (1) the interpretation may be incorrect, (2) the patient may not be ready for it, and (3) the patient is prevented from having the opportunity to achieve the insight on his own. And as Sullivan notes, "The supply of interpretations, like that of advice, greatly exceeds the need for them."[41]

19. INTRODUCING AN UNRELATED TOPIC . . . changing the subject.

Patient. I'd like to die.
Nurse. Did you have visitors this week end?

When the nurse changes the subject or introduces one, she takes over the direction of the discussion. The initiative is taken from the patient. The nurse often does this in order to get to something that she wants to discuss or to get away from a topic that she would prefer not to discuss. Sometimes she just feels the need to say something. Whatever the reason, she usually ends up directing the discussion in all but the most fruitful channels. Schwartz and Shockley recommend that the nurse keep herself open and free to hear the patient, to take in all that is being conveyed. She not only receives the patient's communication but listens to the thoughts and feelings aroused in her for clues that they might give her in understanding the patient. She tries to visualize herself in the patient's place in order to hear him better. This process involves receptivity on the part of the nurse, who waits for the patient's communication, follows his leads, and takes her cue from him instead of directing the communicative situation.[42]

Wolberg[43] states:

Studies of the learning process show that the most effective learning occurs when the individual is concerned with things of strong emotional significance.

[37] Rogers, *op. cit.*, p. 31.
[38] Matheney and Topalis, *op. cit.*, p. 90.
[39] Rogers, Carl R.: *Counseling and Psychotherapy*. Boston: Houghton Mifflin, 1942, p. 196.
[40] Brammer and Shostrom, *op. cit.*, p. 260.
[41] Sullivan, Harry Stack: *Conceptions of Modern Psychiatry,* 2nd ed. New York: Norton, 1953, p. 187.
[42] Schwartz and Shockley, *op. cit.*, pp. 235–36.
[43] Wolberg, Lewis R.: *The Technique of Psychotherapy*. New York: Grune and Stratton, 1954, pp. 165–66.

Discussing material of no immediate interest to the patient interferes with learning. This is why the therapist must sensitize himself to current emotions and trends and not throw the patient off by introducing irrelevant topics or asking unrelated questions.

There are other discontinuities in the discussion that are nurse-introduced. Bachand has defined six "problematic verbal patterns," each with a number of subcategories, by which student nurses in their initial interviews with psychiatric patients avoided problem-centered data. The Bachand PVP Tool, reproduced on page 38, is included so that the reader may recognize other commonly used nontherapeutic techniques that may hinder the patient's learning. Although some of these have already been mentioned—advising, reassuring, interpreting, agreeing—others will warrant the nurse's careful consideration.[44]

[44] Bachand, Joan: *Problematic Verbal Patterns of Student Nurses in Initial Interviews with Psychiatric Patients: A Tool and Its Application.* Master's Thesis, College of Nursing, Rutgers–The State University of New Jersey, 1959.

INTERPERSONAL TECHNIQUES

NONTHERAPEUTIC TECHNIQUES	EXAMPLES
1. *Reassuring*	I wouldn't worry about. . . . Everything will be all right. You're coming along fine.
2. *Giving Approval*	That's good. I'm glad that you. . . .
3. *Rejecting*	Let's not discuss. . . . I don't want to hear about. . . .
4. *Disapproving*	That's bad. I'd rather you wouldn't. . . .
5. *Agreeing*	That's right. I agree.
6. *Disagreeing*	That's wrong. I definitely disagree with. . . . I don't believe that.
7. *Advising*	I think you should. . . . Why don't you. . . ?
8. *Probing*	Now tell me about. . . . Tell me your life history.
9. *Challenging*	But how can you be President of th United States? If you're dead, why is your heart bea ing?

NONTHERAPEUTIC TECHNIQUES	EXAMPLES
0. *Testing*	What day is this? Do you know what kind of a hospital this is? Do you still have the idea that. . . ?
1. *Defending*	This hospital has a fine reputation. No one here would lie to you. But Dr. B. is a very able psychiatrist. I'm sure that he has your welfare in mind when he. . . .
2. *Requesting an Explanation*	Why do you think that? Why do you feel this way? Why did you do that?
3. *Indicating the Existence of an External Source*	What makes you say that? Who told you that you were Jesus? What made you do that?
4. *Belittling Feelings Expressed*	**Patient.** I have nothing to live for . . . I wish I was dead. **Nurse.** Everybody gets down in the dumps. **or** I've felt that way sometimes.
15. *Making Stereotyped Comments*	Nice weather we're having. I'm fine, and how are you? It's for your own good. Keep your chin up. Just listen to your doctor and take part in activities—you'll be home in no time.
16. *Giving Literal Responses*	**Patient.** I'm an Easter egg. **Nurse.** What shade? **or** You don't look like one. **Patient.** They're looking in my head with television. **Nurse.** Try not to watch television. **or** With what channel?
17. *Using Denial*	**Patient.** I'm nothing. **Nurse.** Of course you're something. Everybody is somebody. **Patient.** I'm dead. **Nurse.** Don't be silly.
18. *Interpreting*	What you really mean is. . . . Unconsciously you're saying. . . .
19. *Introducing an Unrelated Topic*	**Patient.** I'd like to die. **Nurse.** Did you have visitors this weekend?

BACHAND PVP TOOL* FOR ANALYZING INTERVIEW RESPONSES OF THE NURSE FOLLOWING NURSE-PATIENT RELATIONSHIP SESSIONS

	INTERVIEW SESSIONS							
	1	*2*	*3*	*4*	*5*	*6*	*7*	*Total*
I. *Switches off problem-centered data by talking about:*								
a. Unrelated focus								
b. Incidental material								
II. *Maintains superficial discussion by:*								
a. Elaboration								
b. Switch to unrelated superficial focus								
III. *Intervenes personally by:*								
a. Giving opinion to life situation of patient without exploring								
b. Giving unsolicited personal opinion to nonpersonal topic								
c. Giving personal information								
d. Complimenting or flattering								
e. Moralizing								
f. Seeking agreement from the patient on opinion								
IV. *Closes off exploration by:*								
a. Prematurely giving an interpretation								
b. Prematurely advising solutions								
c. Prematurely giving reassurance								
V. *Introduces or follows illogical content by:*								
a. Changing key words without validating change								
b. Following vague content or referent as if understood								
c. Introducing vague content or referent								
d. Questioning on different topics or levels without awaiting reply								
e. Speaking to question or statement of patient in conflicting ways								
f. Ignoring question of patient								
VI. *Reinforces pathology by:*								
a. Directly opposing stated belief or feeling of patient								
b. Agreeing with autistic inventions of patient								
c. Agreeing with self-devaluations or projections of patient								
Total times problematic verbal patterns were used in each session: Pattern I								
Pattern II								
Pattern III								
Pattern IV								
Pattern V								
Pattern VI								

Use of the Tool
1. Identify each nurse response;
2. Mark it NP (Nonproblematic) or P (Problematic);
3. Place P responses using tool;
4. Total.

(Nonproblematic response of the nurse is one that maintains focus and aids learning.)

* Bachand, Joan: *Problematic Verbal Patterns of Student Nurses in Initial Interviews with Psychiatric Patients: A Tool and Its Application.* Master's Thesis. College of Nursing. Rutgers–The State University of New Jersey. 1959.

II

Illustrative Clinical Material

Study 1. *MR. JOHN H.* ______

A Relationship with a Hostile Patient

The patient, aged 22, is one of 12 children, of whom eight are now living. The family moved often. The parents are said to have been neglectful. The oldest brother has a prison record; two sisters have been illegitimately pregnant; another sister is mentally retarded and has never attended school. When the patient was nine years old, the father deserted the family. At 10 years, the patient began to be truant from school. He was placed in a disciplinary class at 14 and a year later was sent to a school for difficult and disturbed Negro boys. In less than six months he ran away. He returned to public school and at 16 was dropped as "uneducable." After a series of odd jobs, he enlisted, at 18, in the Marine Corps. He did well there until the onset of his illness nine months later in Japan. His hospitalization followed a four-day period of amnesia. He was sent to a naval hospital in the United States and in three months was sent to a Veterans Administration hospital, where he has spent the last two years.

First Week

MONDAY

N[1]–1. Good morning. [*Greeting.*]

P[2]–2. Good morning. (The nurse sat down beside the patient. She had told him that she would be seeing him each day.)

P–3. What do you want to know?

N–4. We'll talk about whatever you want to talk about. [*Giving broad opening. "We" should be avoided. It tends to build dependency, tying*

[1] Nurse.
[2] Patient.

nurse and patient together. "You can talk about whatever is of concern to you."]

P–5. Talk! I thought you wanted the facts about why I'm in here—why they won't let me go home.

N–6. We can talk about that if you want. [*Accepting. By eliminating "if you want," the risk of his choosing not to talk about it is lessened.*]

P–7. Well—I think why they're keeping me in here—they dislike me and everyone I associate with. The only peace I get is when I go to bed—that's the only time I can get any rest, without anybody haunting me.

N–8. Why do they hate you, John? [*Requesting an explanation. Perhaps she could restate, instead, "You feel disliked—hated even," or encourage description of perceptions, "What happens that prevents you from resting?" "Why" questions are very intimidating.*]

P–9. I don't say they hate me—they dislike me—'cause I'm wiser than they are. I ain't done nothing to them; I try to get along with them. They ain't my people. I don't think I ever seen any of them before. They're strange. And I'm wise of what they're planning.

N–10. How do you mean they're "strange"? [*Focusing. Seeking consensual validation. Better worded,* "What *was strange?" "How" asks for the process; "what" asks for description, for content.*]

P–11. They don't listen when I talk to them and they don't understand. They mustn't be my people that realize the facts. I can't understand them. I never came up against people like that till I got into service. I try to put it in my language—Indian—so that they don't understand. 'Cause if they get too wise, anything can happen then. I'm fond of life myself.

N–12. It started when you were in the service? [*Attempting to place the event in time.*]

P–13. Not in service—just when I came to the hospital. The service was great. These people don't act like Americana. My mother, she know what happening. She got forces on the lookout as to what is happening in this hospital to me. Indians is pretty smart, but sometimes they can mess you Indians up too.

N–14. You're an Indian? [*Voicing doubt.*]

P–15. Yeh.

N–16. I didn't know that. [*Indicating absence of such information in an attempt to reinforce the expression of doubt.*]

P–17. Cherokee. My records say Negro, but my father is an Indian. I'm supposed to follow him—like father, like son. If this keeps on, I have to get in touch with this certain person. They would be destroyed. I got to make sure I get the right person. Everybody is different. Nobody is the same. You understand your own nationality. I'm going to begin from the start—when I came here from San Diego, they wised me up as to what would happen.

N–18. Who told you what would happen? [*Seeking clarification, trying to identify "they."*]

P–19. I can't say that. I can't talk about that. The information get in the wrong hands—it might backfire. I ain't saying you don't understand me, but you might let it slip. I keep it quiet. To tell you the truth, I'm Marine Corps all the way through. That's all I know. (Pause.)

P–20. Now unless you want to talk about my personal life, that's all I know. You got to be careful these days; I learned that in the service. I know facts 'cause I'm an Indian. But they don't know, and I'm not going to wise them up.

N–21. But you have some special knowledge? [*Focusing. Verbalizing the implied.*]

P–22. Knowledge?

N–23. Things other people don't know? [*Clarifying.*]

P–24. I'll put it like this—let's say I got more functions than they got.

N–25. Special senses? [*Seeking consensual validation of "functions."*]

P–26. No, certain kind of person know what happen, what going to happen.

N–27. You know what's going to happen in the future? [*Seeking clarification.*]

P–28. No, what's happening now. I'm keeping it from happening to America, 'cause it's my world as much as anybody else's.

N–29. You mean something could happen to this country? [*Restating. "You mean" is better omitted.*]

P–30. Not country. World!

N–31. Something bad, you mean? [*Verbalizing the implied—to ascertain whether the patient is saying what she thinks he is. "Something bad, you're saying?" would be less intimidating.*]

P–32. Not bad. Could be bad if you don't keep it from happening some way.

N–33. Could you tell me more about it? [*Exploring.*]

P–34. Well, it's like this—at a certain time, a certain day, it happens. But I got ways of stopping it. I got someone else working with me, but we keep it secret.

N–35. Somebody here working with you? [*Seeking clarification—to find out whether he feels that he has any allies in the hospital or whether everyone seems to be against him.*]

P–36. No. It's this whole hospital. We got them running, fighting—'cause we do the fighting, the killing. You kill them or they kill you.

N–37. This whole hospital is working against you? [*Restating. Frequent restatement seems indicated since he often appears to contradict himself.*]

P–38. No—every time they do something, it backfires on them. There got to be someone big behind it, and I am one of them. [*He seems to be saying that everyone in the hospital is working against him, but ineffectively.*]

N–39. There's a whole group of you then? [*Restating.*]

P–40. There's millions—millions of warriors.

N–41. What exactly are you fighting against? [*Exploring.*]

P–42. It's not exactly enemy. They talking a little too much about the world, and they don't know about life. It might destroy the world, and I one of the persons got to keep it going. It's my job.

N–43. How did you get this job? [*Encouraging description of perceptions. Perhaps better worded, "What led up to your getting this job?"*]

P–44. Through signals and people telling me what to do—that's how I know what's happening in the world. If anything slips, they might kill me—my own people. And I don't want to die. I be on the right side.

N–45. This is a tough situation to be in, isn't it? [*Attempting to translate into feelings.*]

P–46. Depends on how you look at it. You be on the right—the right always wins.

N–47. But you have to fight all these people. [*Verbalizing the implied. The nurse is asking, "Is this how it seems?"*]

P–48. I don't have to fight them. Oh, occasionally I might slip and knock one of them on his can. If he's on the wrong side, I got to change his mind.

N–49. How can you tell when they're on the wrong side—an enemy? [*Encouraging description of perceptions. "How" asks for process rather than content. Better worded, "What is it that indicates when they're on the wrong side?"*]

P–50. You can tell by how they walk, how they look. It's easy. They don't belong in our world.

N–51. Are some here in the hospital? [*Exploring.*]

P–52. Oh yes, but they wasn't here from the start—they weren't here in our world. I don't know what world they came from.

N–53. And they're trying to destroy our world? [*Restating—to be sure this is what he is saying.*]

P–54. They're trying, but they won't succeed. That's what I'm for, and others who love America.

N–55. Some of the people here are on your side? [*Seeking clarification of "others." Perhaps if she just asks, "The others?" the response will be more informative. This point is worthy of further exploration.*]

P–56. No, none of them. They strange.

N–57. They're all from another world? [*Restating—for her own understanding.*]

P–58. They're not from our world.

N–59. Where did they come from? [*Exploring.*]

P–60. I don't know. I know, but it just didn't come to me yet. But if you come back every day, I think I'll find that out from them—'cause America is strong.

(He sank into his chair and closed his eyes.)

N–61. It must be lonely—with all these strange people. [*Attempting to translate into feelings. The patient has just indicated his interest in the relationship being a continuing one. The nurse seeks to convey that she is aware of his loneliness and aloneness with his problems.*]

P–62. You can say that! I miss my own people.

TUESDAY

P–1. It's like this—I don't think I need help.

N–2. I thought I could understand how you feel. [*Offering self. Better worded, "Tell me more about this" or "What are your feelings?" To use the word "understand" is to imply that the nurse is grasping for an inference, an abstraction, a classification of the problem. The nurse must do this for herself, but in the relationship it is more useful to let the patient know that for some time the effort is to get what is said, to hear, to follow, and, when such data are fully collected, for both nurse and patient to try to grasp the significance of the raw data, i.e., to understand what the data were about.*[3]]

P–3. It ain't hard. It's easy 'cause it's normal—sensible. It's easy to catch on and understand.

N–4. That's what I'm trying to do. [*Offering self.*]

P–5. Well, understanding is great—if you understand what I'm talking about. I believe in putting the facts to you straight. You come every day, I'll explain it to you. It's hard to understand what I'm talking about—it's the way I live. It takes time. I think you'll catch on to it. [*The patient's*

[3] Peplau, Hildegard E.: personal communication to the authors, May, 1962.

reply seems to support the idea that understanding will require much time and effort.]

N–6. That's why I write it down—so I get it straight. [*Giving information about role of the notebook.*]

(Patient laughed.)

N–7. Not used to people writing down what you say? [*Tentatively suggesting meaning for the anxious laughter.*]

P–8. Oh yeh, I'm used to it—it happen. Well, things happen in this world that you got to face. You got to be wise—to keep up to what they doing to destroy the world.

N–9. Why do they want to destroy it? [*Requesting an explanation. He actually does not know. Perhaps "they" have to destroy it so that he can save it. In other words, there has to be "'evil" for him to overcome so that he can prove himself. The patient, of course, is not aware that these are the probable dynamics involved; and the nurse understands that such interpretations would have little or no therapeutic value, especially this early in the relationship. Perhaps he will, at some time, come to this conclusion, or a similar one, on his own, after he learns much more about himself and his relationships with others.*]

P–10. I think you know that. Everybody fight for what they believe in. And I'm on the side of right all the way. I guess if this keeps up, seem like there won't be no hope—unless I do my best at a certain time and make good over that power of the enemy. Well, that's it. (Pause.) I guess I'll get some water. I'll be right back. (He returned.) What else do you want to know—how I like my eggs? Well done.

N–11. We can talk about whatever's important to you. [*Giving broad opening. "You and I" is preferable to "we."*]

P–12. Important to me?

N–13. Yes. [*Reaffirming what she has said. He seems surprised that someone is interested.*]

P–14. In my life, nothing's important to me, except my mother. I love her. I guess everyone love their mother. I know I do.

N–15. Nothing else is important? [*Restating. The nurse could have followed up his comment and explored further the relationship with his mother.*]

P–16. Yeh, my sisters and brothers, nieces and nephews.

N–17. Sounds as though you have a pretty nice family. [*Giving approval. Perhaps she could restate, "They—and your mother—are important to you."*]

P–18. Oh, yeh, I hope so, for my sake.

N–19. You mean they're with you all the way. [*Verbalizing the implied. The nurse voices what she thinks he is saying. Actually he didn't put it quite this positively.*]

P–20. The family stick together—that's the way it is.

N–21. But nobody else understands. [*Verbalizing the implied.*]

P–22. I don't know no more—that's all there is to it.

N–23. You don't have to talk all the time I'm here. [*Giving information about his role in the relationship.*]

P–24. I'm done talking.

(He got up and paced about the room. He danced a bit to the music on the radio, shadowboxed, sat down, laughed, then looked serious.)

N–25. I'll be leaving in a few minutes. [*Giving information. This prepared the patient for the nurse's leaving. Otherwise, he might feel that she left because he was not talking with her.*]

(He nodded, got up, walked around the room, looked in the mirror, rubbed his hand through his hair, and returned.)

N–26. I'll see you tomorrow. [*Giving information.*]

P–27. Okay, see you tomorrow.

WEDNESDAY

P–1. I'm not talking today.

N–2. Okay. Do you want to tell me why? [*Accepting. Requesting an explanation. She might say, "You don't feel like talking today."*]

P–3. I just ain't talking.

N–4. You don't have to talk if you don't want to. [*Giving information about his role. "If you don't want to" is better omitted. The tone would be less negative.*]

N–5. Do you mind if I stay here? [*Offering self. Encouraging evaluation. She could be more direct and ask whether it would make him uncomfortable if she stayed.*]

P–6. No, you can stay.

(There was a long pause. He got up to get a light from a nursing assistant, occasionally laughing inappropriately. He looked up at the television briefly several times, looked directly at the nurse once, laughing uncomfortably, then held his head in his hands. His group was called for occupational therapy. In the shop he paced back and forth.)

N–7. May I walk with you? [*Offering self.*]

P–8. Sure, if you want to.

N–9. Do you feel better when you're walking? [*Encouraging evaluation. Perhaps this could be asked in a way that would require more than a "yes" or "no" response.*]

P–10. Sure.

(About 15 minutes passed during which the patient and the nurse paced back and forth.)

P–11. Getting tired. Want to sit down?

N–12. It's up to you. [*Reflecting. Allowing the patient to decide.*]

(He returned to the table. Patient and nurse sat together in silence until it was time for her to leave.)

THURSDAY

N–1. Good morning, John. [*Offering recognition.*]

P–2. Good morning.

(The patient was pacing.)

N–3. Would you like to sit down awhile? [*Tentatively suggesting action.*]

P–4. No, I'm walking.

(In a few moments he came and sat by the nurse.)

N–5. Anything you'd like to talk about this morning? [*Offering broad opening.*]

(He shook his head "no." He left, then returned.)

N–6. I'm interested in trying to understand how you feel—to try to help you. [*Offering self. Perhaps better worded, "I'm interested in your feelings" or "I'd like to know what your feelings are."*]

(He shook his head "no" again and walked away. He returned shortly.)

P–7. Now! What would you like to know?

N–8. Whatever you'd like to tell me—whatever will help me understand you. [*Giving broad opening, as well as information about her role. Better worded, "Whatever will help me be aware of your feelings."*]

P–9. I loved a woman once. She was pretty, but she put me down.

N–10. For someone else? [*Verbalizing the implied.*]

(He nodded.)

N–11. How did that make you feel? [*Encouraging evaluation. Rather than ask "how," the nurse could say, "What were your feelings when this happened?"*]

P–12. When that clock strikes 11:30, watch for something to happen.

N–13. I won't be here then. [*Giving information.*]

P–14. When you going?

N–15. 9:30. [*Giving information.*]

N–16. Can you tell me what's going to happen? [*Encouraging description of perceptions.*]

P–17. It's pretty hard. It's like this—when a person is after a certain thing and can't reach it, I'm going to see that he don't. It's my will power. That's all!

(He left and walked about the dayroom. He seemed unable to discuss his ideas any further. The nurse spoke as he passed her.)

N–18. Would you like to play a game of Ping-pong? [*Tentatively suggesting action.*]

P–19. Please.

(During the game, which he won 22-20, he kept score and erred frequently as to which one of them had earned the point. His group was then called for a walk. The nurse accompanied him. At one point he sat down on the ground.)

P–20. I can't help laughing.

N–21. About what? [*Offering general lead.*]

P–22. That I'm God—and no one else knows it.

FRIDAY

(The patient brought out a letter, showing his name "John Henry H." He asked the nurse to write down "H. H.")

N–1. What would you like me to call you? [*Seeking clarification.*]

P–2. You can call me H.

N–3. Is there something you'd like to talk about? You said if I came back each day you'd explain things so that I could understand. [*Giving broad opening and restating what he'd said previously. "So that I could understand" could be omitted.*]

N–4. I'd really like to understand. [*Offering self. It would be better to encourage description at this point.*]

P–5. Really ain't much to tell now. So that's how it began—I fell in love from first sight.

N–6. And then? [*Offering general lead.*]

P–7. And then I said—like this—"let me have peace, my friends."

N–8. Peace from what? [*Exploring.*]

(He left, paced, returned.)

P–9. What else do you want to know?

N–10. Whatever will help you. [*Giving broad opening. But he is not* *likely to know what will help him. She could say, "Whatever is of concern to you."*]

P–11. I'd like to talk about love.

(He read over the notes of the above discussion, left, and paced some more.)

P–12. Everyone. I know I'd get them! They ain't going to bother me no more. I killed them. Logical. Twelve of them. They did me some wrong in the future.

(To the nurse)

P–13. It's logical to get revenge, isn't it?

N–14. Why are they against you? [*Requesting an explanation. She might say, "You're angry now and want revenge," or "someone seems about to do you wrong?"*]

P–15. Oh me, here we go again—another one.

(He walked away again. He seemed to be referring to someone or something he "saw" in the room. He held out his hand to the nurse.)

N–16. Friends. [*Accepting. Verbalizing the implied.*]

P–17. Sure.

(He shook the nurse's hand. He then took the notebook and wrote, "I love you, but you got to listle." He apparently meant "listen.")

N–18. I'm here as a nurse to try to help you, so that you can go home. [*Giving information to clarify her role. The nurse may be setting unrealistic goals when she says, ". . . so that you can go home."*]

P–19. Where is my home?

N–20. I don't know. You never told me. It's with your mother, isn't it? [*Indicating lack of information. Suggesting a possibility.*]

P–21. No.

N–22. Do you want to tell me? [*Reflecting.*]

P–23. I can't tell you that.

Second Week

MONDAY

(The patient had been given an intramuscular injection of chlorpromazine. He slept through the hour. The nurse sat beside him until it was time to leave. Later that morning the nurse saw the patient on the enclosed porch as she was leaving the building. She waved.)

N–1. I see you're awake. [*Making an observation.*]

P–2. (Shouting.) Tell them why you lied!

N–3. I don't think that I did. What did I say? [*Tentatively disagreeing. Encouraging description of perceptions.*]

P–4. I want you to tell them.

(He seemed unable to elaborate and appeared quite disturbed and angry. Unfortunately, the nurse had no opportunity to clarify what had occurred.)

TUESDAY

(The patient was receiving neutral pack therapy in the hydrotherapy room.)

P–1. Tell them why you lied!!

N–2. I haven't lied to you, H. [*Disagreeing. The patient cannot be reasoned with. The nurse might say, "You believe that I lied to you about something," or "What happened that gave you this impression?"*]

P–3. Tell them why you lied!!

N–4. Tell me what I said. [*Encouraging description of perceptions.*]

P–5. Tell them that you want to kill me!!

N–6. I don't want to hurt you—I want to help you. [*Disagreeing. Telling him this is unlikely to be effective. She might state, "You feel that I want to harm you."*]

P–7. Tell them the truth—tell them I am God. Tell them you wanted me instead of your husband. And I don't want you.

N–8. I'm here as a nurse to help you—that's the only reason. [*Giving information. It would appear that he felt the nurse was getting too close to him emotionally, possibly arousing sexual feelings that he must now project onto her.*]

P–9. You destroyed them—my brothers and sisters and nieces and nephews. They just now died.

N–10. I want to help people live; I don't want anyone to die—that's why I'm a nurse. [*Defending. In defending her own good intentions, the nurse stops seeking to understand his feelings and their origin. Perhaps she could comment, "You feel that I have the power to destroy your family."*]

P–11. Get out! You betrayed your people. Call it off. Tell them the truth—why you want to kill me.

N–12. I don't want to kill you. [*Disagreeing. She might say, "Something has happened to cause you to feel betrayed."*]

P–13. Now go away from me.

N–14. All right. (She stepped back.) If you change your mind, I'll be here awhile. [*Complying, but continuing to offer self.*]

P–15. You destroyed your country. Get the ____ out of here. Still trying to kill God. I'm right here—GOD! [*Perhaps the patient feels that the nurse wants to "kill" or destroy the image that he has created of himself as "God."*]

P–16. I know my mother made it—she always do. Tell them the truth—tell them who lied.

N–17. I don't think anyone lied. You just misunderstand. I'm trying to help you. [*Tentatively disagreeing. Attempting to explain. She might say here, "You feel that the truth is being withheld."*]

N–18. If it helps you to be angry with me, go ahead. [*Offering self. Allowing the expression of negative feelings.*]

P–19. So you want to live. You're not dead?

N–20. No. [*Giving information.*]

P–21. I'm not dead?

N–22. No. [*Giving information.*]

P–23. But why am I in pack?

N–24. To help you relax. [*Giving information.*]

P–25. You want to_____with God. Get the_____out of my face.

N–26. Why are you angry with me? I want to help you. [*Requesting an explanation. Perhaps she could quietly state, "You feel very angry with me now," or "You've somehow gotten the impression that our relationship is no longer on a nurse-patient basis."*]

(He then began to address an illusory figure.)

P–27. Thank you, Brownie, I owe you that much. Shoot them both—those is my orders. Shoot them. That's better. Now put them in pack. Shoot *my* mother—you traitor!

P–28. Don't do it, Brownie.

P–29. Get out of here. I know what you done, you_____. Tell the truth now—why do you want to kill my mother?

N–30. I don't want to kill her. [*Disagreeing. She might say, "Something has happened to give you the notion that I want to harm your mother."*]

P–31. Who's your husband?

N–32. I don't have one. [*Giving information.*]

P–33. Dr. P. is your husband.

N–34. He has a wife of his own. [*Giving information.*]

P–35. Don't get her now, Brownie. Let Dr. P. take her out.

P–36. You lie and we're coming after you—me and my warriors. It ain't seven yet. It come seven and you have your walk. Look who betray your country. That _____.

P–37. Now you want forgiveness for betraying your God. Betraying my country. You better kill me 'cause I get out of this pack I'm going to kill you!

(It was time for the patient to come out of pack. The nurse waited in the dayroom until he showered and dressed. He came into the room but sat far from the nurse. Then he paced about, at times quietly, at other times cursing. The nurse told him that it was time for her to leave. His response consisted of demands for her to go and more cursing.)

WEDNESDAY

N–1. Good morning. [*Greeting.*]

(The patient did not reply but came to where the nurse was sitting.)

P–2. Got a cigarette?

(The nurse gave him a cigarette and a light.)

P–3. I'll be back.

N–4. Okay. [*Accepting.*]

(He returned.)

P–5. I said that I love you, right?

N–6. Did you say that? [*Reflecting.*]

P–7. Yes. Do you love me?

N–8. I like you. I like lots of people. I'm here as a nurse to help you get well and go home. [*Giving approval. Making a stereotyped comment. Giving information. She might say, "I respect you as a person and care about your well-being." She might even add, "What kind of love did you have in mind?"*]

(He read over the notes.)

P–9. Good.

(He put out his hand.)

N–10. Friends? [*Verbalizing the implied.*]

(The patient shook the nurse's hand.)

P–11. Never tell, never tell.

N–12. What do you mean? [*Seeking clarification. "Mean" tends to be intimidating. The nurse could say, "Tell me in greater detail—I don't follow you."*]

P–13. I'm not talking. You know what I mean.

N–14. I'm not sure that I do know what you mean. [*Indicating need for further clarification.*]

P–15. I'll be back.

N–16. Okay. [*Accepting.*]

(He walked about. While looking straight ahead he said—)

P–17. Go ahead, kill me. I'm the enemy, here I am.

N–18. Who are you talking to? [*Seeking clarification.*]

P–19. I'm talking to whoever is concerned.

N–20. I'm trying to understand, John. You said you'd help. [*Offering self. Restating what he'd said previously. Description should be encouraged. "Will you tell me more about it?"*]

P–21. Why did you put your husband down?

N–22. I don't have a husband. (Showing him her left hand.) [*Giving information.*]

P–23. Do you know Dr. P.?

N–24. Yes, to say hello to. He's on Building 12. [*Giving information.*]

P–25. When you going to tell the truth? Why did you tell them where my village was—so that they could destroy my people?

N–26. I didn't tell them. I don't know where your village is. [*Indicating absence of such information. But this is a rather literal response. It seems to imply that "they" are known to the nurse and that a "village" exists. Perhaps she could merely say, "I have no knowledge of such a village."*]

P–27. You don't know where my Indian village is?

N–28. No. You never told me. [*Giving information.*]

P–29. Good.
(He read over the notes.)

P–30. Tell them why you want to kill my brother—you and all of them.

N–31. I'm on your side. [*Giving a literal response. The nurse presumably means to imply only that she is not aligned against him. The patient may well interpret the comment to mean that she is literally taking sides—an acknowledgment that the "enemy" is real.*]

P–32. We'll see.
(He left and returned.)

P–33. So you don't know where my Indian village is.

N–34. No. [*Indicating lack of information. She might word it, "I know of no Indian village."*]

P–35. I'll tell you.
(The patient spoke unintelligibly, presumably in "Cherokee" or his version of the language.)

N–36. I don't understand. [*Seeking clarification. Perhaps better worded, "I don't follow you."*]

P–37. Over there—down the hill.

N–38. Down the hill? [*Restating.*]

P–39. Yes. Do you want war or peace?

N–40. What do you want? [*Reflecting.*]

P–41. I would like to have peace. Now what do you want?

N–42. I'd like to have peace. [*Giving a literal response that implies a "war" does in fact exist. Perhaps she could merely state, "Peace seems preferable to war," or "You seem to feel that there is no further need for fighting, is that correct?"*]

P–43. Okay, then stop the war. I don't want to hurt your people or you mine.

N–44. Okay. [*Accepting. The nurse implies that she can "stop the war." She might restate, "There is to be no further conflict; no one is to be hurt."*]

(The patient then spoke in the direction of an imaginary figure.)

P–45. Sitting Bull, you lie. Now you die.

(He made the gesture of "shooting" Sitting Bull.)

P–46. Tell them why they killed my brothers. Tell the truth. They killed them. I saw it on TV.

N–47. I didn't know about it. [*Indicating lack of information. Perhaps exploration is indicated here. The nurse might say, "On television? How could that be? Could you tell me more about it?"*]

P–48. I'm taking revenge for my brothers and sisters.

N–49. On TV they're just acting. [*Attempting to present reality. Further description would seem worthwhile at this time. The nurse could ask, "Just exactly what happened? I don't follow you."*]

P–50. Well, I'm not acting. I'm killing to revenge my brothers and sisters. Tell them why they killed my brothers and sisters. They're your friends. You kill my people, I kill yours and then you. [*Perhaps the nurse did not have time to reply. It would have been well if she had. Such strong comments of feeling should not seem to be ignored. She might accept his feelings by stating, "You've come to believe that your family has been killed, and you are very angry."*]

(The patient's group was escorted to the occupational therapy shop. There he asked the nurse—)

P–51. Who am I? What is my name?

N–52. I thought it was John Henry H. [*Giving information.*]

P–53. That's it. That's right.

P–54. I was alive at first—wasn't never dead. They tried to kill me, but got the wrong man—stabbing them, killing them—but they never got me. I must be the leader. They never get my mother or my father either. They must be after somebody big. If I find him, I'm going to give him to them. My warriors deserve that. These psychiatrists is after God, isn't they?

N–55. They are? [*Perhaps she might add, "What has happened to give you that impression?"*]

P–56. Sure, didn't you know that?

N–57. I didn't think they were. [*Tentatively disagreeing. Instead, she could voice doubt by commenting, "That seems unusual," or "That would be strange." She might also ask, "What events have led you to that conclusion?" He may feel that the psychiatrists are trying to "kill" or destroy his identification with God.*]

P–58. Everyone I see I kill them.

(He made another "shooting" gesture in the direction of an imaginary figure who "drew" on him.)

N–59. It's time for me to leave now. I'll see you tomorrow. [*Giving information.*]

THURSDAY

(When the nurse entered the dayroom, the patient was playing Ping-pong with another patient. John told this patient that he [John] was God and that Dr. P. was his father. He then greeted the nurse and found two seats for them.)

N–1. What's this about Dr. P.? [*Seeking clarification.*]

P–2. Isn't he your husband?

N–3. No. [*Giving information.*]

P–4. Aren't you my mother?

N–5. No. [*Giving information.*]

P–6. Who are you? What's your name?

N–7. Miss S. I'm a nurse. [*Giving information.*]

P–8. You got nice hands.

(He walked out onto the enclosed porch. There he shouted loudly something about being "agin 'em." He returned and asked the nurse to play Ping-pong with him. A game was begun.)

P–9. You're my star. You with me to the end?

N–10. Yes. [*Offering self. It would seem, however, that the nurse and the patient have two entirely different ideas in mind here.*]

P–11. Then I with you to the end. I love you.

(The patient stopped playing Ping-pong abruptly, walked about, and then postured with his arm extended as though he were a gunman. He addressed an imaginary person.)

P–12. Draw your gun. I got mine.

(He then "shot," after which he returned to the nurse.)

P–13. We talk now.

(He escorted the nurse to a chair.)

N–14. Who were you shooting? [*Exploring. A bit too literal. Perhaps better worded, "What was happening there? You acted as though you thought you were shooting someone."*]

P–15. Seems like I got my man—now there's one more. Not man, it's supposed to be a woman.

(He walked away. There was more "shooting." Then he spoke to another patient.)

P–16. Nine o'clock, I'm going to kill you. I'm God—H.—see? You better draw, 'cause even if you don't I'm going to kill you. I'm taking revenge, see. Nine o'clock. From the Russians on D day—I kept the peace. You wanted to bomb the Russians too. Walk right into that knife. You didn't know the Indians would track you down, did you?

(The nurse told him that she would see him the next day.)

P–17. Wait till you see this shooting. (He "shot.")

P–18. I'll see you tomorrow. You tell the truth, I'll tell the truth.

N–19. Right. [*Accepting.*]

(He then told the nurse not to lie any more, that he had proof that she lied. He pulled out a dead flower and said that it was proof.)

FRIDAY

P–1. Tell them that I'm God. They're trying to kill God. They tried to electrocute me day before yesterday, but they got the wrong man.

N–2. But you want peace. [*Restating comment of several days ago. It does not seem too appropriate at this time. Perhaps she could respond, "You feel that someone is trying to kill you."*]

P–3. No peace—war! After what they done, I want war. I never killed a man, but I'm going to kill one now and more and more.

P–4. Got a match, please?

N–5. Sure. [*Complying with request.*]

P–6. Tell them that's high explosive and I could destroy the world. But I'm protecting the world and the peoples in it. Tell them I took a chance with my life to save those scoundrels. I don't want them near me no more. My brother and I stick together. We track them down.

(He read over the notes.)

P–7. What kind of writing is that? Latin?

N–8. English. [*Giving a literal response. Perhaps she could ask, "Does it seem strange?"*]

P–9. You English?

N–10. No, I'm American. [*Giving information.*]

P–11. American? Okay. We don't want war, but if they poison my peoples, we will take revenge and kill them. My brother and me will kill them all.

I kept the peace for so long that I'm getting tired of keeping it. If they want war, we'll give them one. That's it. I got plenty more where they came from. My brother and I can destroy them any time we want. No more talk. That's it. Tell them they keep on trying to fool God, but they don't fool me a bit. They want war, I give them war—if they want it.

[*The nurse has assumed the role of an interested listener. The patient seems more concerned with making his point than with receiving any response from the nurse. He seems to feel that her notes will communicate his ideas to others. He prefaces most of his remarks with "tell them" as though others will read the comments.*]

Tell them that Black Cloud lied to tell truth. What's behind it? Tell them—why do they do things crazy sometimes and blame it on me, Chief Running Cloud? Tell them I'm ready to fight and die for my country. They don't know that there's a war on. They bombed the Russians and now they're trying to hurt me. But I'm not going to let them hurt me—I got high explosives. Tell them that they failed. But when I get ready for war, I'll get out there with them and fight. Tell them that they tried to destroy my world, but I outsmarted them. Tell them they don't know Chief Running Cloud know everything. Tell them they can't outsmart me no way, shape, or form.

Just keep on playing with God and see what happens. He was a good God but they changed him. You want war, you get war. The next time this happens I'm ready to fight, if they keep on stirring up trouble.

I'm trying to save people's lives. I been doing it all my life. They are turning against God. I always stand up for my rights. I ain't afraid of nothing. Tell them that I like a guy once, but it seemed like he don't understand. But I give him time to make up his mind whose side he's on before I kill him. And I don't want to do that because I like him. That's all. Tell them that I'm going to kill a man and it won't be hard, 'cause he keep on messing with me. And I'm going to take his scalp—real soon. I just now took his scalp. Tell them a man just drawed on me, and I beat him to the draw.

(When the time was up, the nurse told the patient that she would see him on Monday. Later in the day, during group activity, the patient approached the nurse.)

P–12. Who am I?

N–13. John Henry H. [*Giving information.*]

P–14. What's my other name?

N–15. That's the only name I know. [*Presenting reality. The nurse feels that the patient wanted her to say that he was "God." This she could not do. As a result of this conversation the nurse noted, "It would seem today that the patient has accepted me—if not as a part of his world, at least as a means of communication between himself and others."*]

Third Week

MONDAY

N–1. Good morning, H. [*Giving recognition.*]

P–2. What's new?

N–3. Nothing much. How about you? [*Making stereotyped comments, during which nothing is communicated. This might be an opportune moment for the nurse to restate her role and the purpose of their relationship. She could begin, "I've been wondering whether you fully understand why we are talking together each day."*]

P–4. Naw.

N–5. Have any visitors this week end? [*Introducing a topic for discussion, not leaving the initiative to the patient.*]

P–6. My mother.

N–7. Anything you'd like to talk about today? [*Giving a broad opening and returning the initiative to him.*]

P–8. No, I'm not much for talking.

N–9. You don't have to talk if you don't want to. [*Accepting, giving information about his role. Perhaps better worded, "It isn't necessary to talk all the time."*]

(There was a period of silence.)

P–10. Well, there ain't much to talk about today. You want to play a game of Ping-pong?

N–11. Sure. [*Accepting. Perhaps the nurse might add, "If this is what you want to do." Such a comment makes it clear that it is the patient's needs that govern the utilization of the hour. The patient should not feel that he has to provide amusement for the nurse.*]

(The patient won the game 22–20.)

P–12. You don't want to play no more. Let's sit down.

N–13. Okay. That was a good game. [*Accepting. Giving approval. Perhaps she could say that it was a "close" game rather than introduce the idea of "good and bad." Also she should not allow to pass uncommented upon his expression of what he believes to be her feelings. If he is correct,* *she might say, "You noticed that I was getting tired" or some such comment. If this is not the case, she might ask, "I wonder what gave you that impression?"*]

P–14. I'll be right back; I want to get some water.

(He returned. He seemed thoughtful but relaxed.)

P–15. Let's sit some place else.

N–16. Okay. [*Accepting.*]

P–17. I say that I God. We're going to dig the graves deep for trying to kill God—20 or 40 times—try to electrocute God. Put that down. Trying to tell me what to do—I'll see to that myself. [Note: *the patient was not now on the electroshock therapy but had received a course of treatments while in a naval hospital. He may have had this in mind when he referred to being "electrocuted" 20 or 40 times.*]

P–18. When will this paper be out? I'd like to know when is you going to print it?

N–19. You want it printed? [*Seeking clarification.*]

P–20. Please. I think you can make it by tomorrow. I know where the paper place is at.

N–21. Where is it? [*Exploring. However, she seems to be evading the patient's misinterpretation of her role. Clarification is needed here.*]

(The patient pointed.)

P–22. The *Bulletin* [newspaper] place.

P–23. Hold it my peoples. Don't fight till I give the word. Go, Brownie.

N–24. Go, Brownie? [*Restating.*]

P–25. Yes, that's my dog. Should be about this high now. He's a big dog—can eat them alive. About 9 or 10 years ago—I'm 22 going on 23 now—I was around 12 or 13, I picked up a dog—a good dog. I found him straying through the streets in _____, Virginia, where my mother and father was born. I raised him. He protected us. Somebody stole him, but I got him back—here he is. I protect him—I God. [*The nurse did not respond here, but if she had, she might have stated, "You want to be strong enough to protect those you love from harm." This is realistic and communicates the nurse's understanding of one of the patient's needs.*]

(He read over the notes.)

P–26. That's good enough.

P–27. Tell them my mother and father is still alive. They ain't fooling nobody. They make fools of themselves. That dog already ate up one man for lying—put that down.

They better be ready to fight when I'm ready. Tell them it's an Indian man's world. They think it's a white man's and colored man's world, but it ain't. Send the lions and the tigers, to see if they're well. And the elephants, too. If they're well, we fight. Chief Running Cloud said that—me. That's my horse, Silver. Chief Running Cloud been fighting all his life.

P–28. That's it. No more.

N–29. Okay. [*Accepting.*]

N–30. See you tomorrow. [*Giving information.*]

P–31. You promise?

N–32. Yes, I promise. [*Reinforcing her previous comment.*]

TUESDAY

N–1. Good morning. [*Greeting.*]

P–2. Eight o'clock. What we going to talk about today?

N–3. Whatever you want. [*Reflecting.*]

P–4. Let's don't talk today. Let's play Ping-pong.

N–5. Okay. [*Accepting. She might restate, "You'd rather play Ping-pong today than use our time to talk about what is of concern to you." This would encourage the patient to evaluate whether this is what he prefers. It also recalls the purpose of the relationship. This is not to imply that the nurse is to try to talk the patient into speaking with her. The purpose is rather to make clear the alternatives. The choice should be his. Or she could comment, "You would rather not talk today." The mere repetition may encourage the patient to explore why he would rather not talk.*]

(Four games were played, all of which were won by the patient. The patient's group was called to occupational therapy. In the shop he walked about quietly for awhile, then let out a loud whoop. His comments seemed to be directed to one of the other patients.)

P–6. You think you playing with God, huh? Just keep on playing and see what happens; you're going to die for that. Nobody play with me and get away with it. H.—me—God. We'll see how brave you is when my warriors get here. You risk the life of everybody in here. Stop playing with me.

None of you are going home, see? You're going to stay in Alcatraz, see? None of you play with me. I always stand up for my rights. Come on, Brownie.

N–7. I have to leave now, H. [*Giving information. It almost seems as if the patient were separating his illness from the relationship.*]

P–8. See you tomorrow, okay.

WEDNESDAY

(The patient was playing a game of Ping-pong with another patient when the nurse entered. He completed the game, then came to sit by her.)

P–1. What's happening this morning?

N–2. Nothing yet that I know of. Is something happening? [*Seeking clarification. The nurse may be taking too literally what is meant merely as a greeting, such as "What's new?"*]

P–3. Let's not talk this morning.

N–4. Okay. [*Accepting. Again, the nurse could say something such as, "You prefer not to talk this morning." Perhaps the patient would be encouraged to explore the problem.*]

(The nurse suggested that they could look at some magazines. The patient declined at first, then suggested that they look at one together. He selected a *McCall's* after searching unsuccessfully for a movie magazine. After they had discussed a few items, he closed the book and returned it to the rack.)

N–5. Want to beat me at a game of Ping-pong? [*Suggesting possible action. It would be interesting to know what might have occurred if the nurse had not taken the initiative in proposing activities. It seems as though the nurse was more uncomfortable with the silence than the patient was.*]

P–6. Naw.

N–7. You're too good at Ping-pong for me to beat. [*Giving approval. Perhaps she might have said he was "more skilled."*]

P–8. Too good?

N–9. Uh hmm. [*Reinforcing her comment.*]

(Thereafter they sat quietly in silence. When his group was called for swimming, the nurse told the patient that she would see him tomorrow.)

P–10. Okay, see you tomorrow.

THURSDAY

(The patient asked for a cigarette. The nurse had none. He commented that the ward was out of his brand of "Indian" cigarettes.)

P–1. Tough.

N–2. What's tough? Not having any cigarettes? [*Seeking clarification.*]

P–3. Life. Life is tough.

N–4. I guess life is tough. [*Accepting.*]

P–5. It's nice—nice if you know how to live it.

N–6. I guess all any of us can do is be ourselves. [*Giving advice, but at the same time implying that being himself is all that is expected of him, that being himself is acceptable, and that, in fact, it is all that he can be.*]

P–7. Yes, be ourselves—that's about it.

N–8. Is it hard to be yourself sometimes? [*Suggesting tentative meaning.*]

P–9. Not for me. Maybe for other patients, but not for me.
(Pause.)

N–10. What are you thinking about? [*Giving broad opening.*]

P–11. Nothing.

N–12. I want to help, if there's any way I can. [*Offering self.*]

P–13. How many times have I heard that—three?

N–14. I don't know. I didn't keep count. [*Indicating lack of information.*]

P–15. I do. It was three or four. Good. (Pause.) [*The nurse's offer seemed to have meaning for him.*]

P–16. Want to play a game of Ping-pong?

N–17. Sure. [*Accepting.*]

(The patient won the game 21–9, keeping score very accurately this time.)

N–18. I have to leave now. It's 9:30. [*Giving information.*]

P–19. See you tomorrow.

N–20. Right. [*Confirming what he has said.*]

P–21. You'll be here tomorrow.

N–22. You bet—eight o'clock. So long. [*Reinforcing her comment.*]

FRIDAY

N–1. Hi.

P–2. Good morning.
(The patient was playing Ping-pong with a nursing assistant.)

N–3. You beat him again? [*Making a tentative observation.*]

P–4. Yep.

N–5. How many games did you win? [*Making social conversation while he is engaged in activity with others.*]

P–6. Seven.

N–7. How many did K. win? [*As above.*]

P–8. None.

N–9. Wow! [*Expressing surprise.*]

(The patient laughed.)

P–10. Too bad.

(He then played a game with one of the patients and won. Medications were called.)

P–11. I'm going to get my medication. I'll be right back.

N–12. Right. [*Accepting.*]

(He then played Ping-pong with another nursing assistant. He looked to the nurse for recognition at times but was also able to compliment his opponents on their good shots. He then sat by the nurse.)

N–13. Care for a Chesterfield? [*Offering a cigarette.*]

P–14. No, I got two packs today.

(They sat in silence for a time. The patient seemed at ease. He began speaking in earnest. The nurse states that she put aside her notebook so that she could react fully to what he said. Later she noted, "He told me that he played Ping-pong to pass the time and to keep busy. He discussed his family, relating the event that produced the death of his two small nephews whom he loved—they had smothered to death in an empty refrigerator in a vacated apartment where they were playing with an older boy. The mother of the boys required hospitalization for awhile at a state hospital, he related, but now is well and has a daughter. He mentioned that his girl friend had written him a letter and that he had seen her on his previous week ends at home 'before she turned me out.' He said that she had a nice handwriting and a good education. He told me about his desire to go home, to take care of his mother, eventually to build her a house, and to establish himself in a job—construction work. He hopes to get back together with his girl friend if possible."

The nurse suggested that he might like to talk with his doctor also about his plans and his desire to work toward going home. The patient told her, in closing, that he had an appointment with the doctor for Monday.)

The nurse continued the relationship with this patient for five more weeks, during which time he gave no further evidence of hallucinations or delusions of being God or an Indian chief. He engaged in games of cards and Ping-pong with the nurse and with others and discussed with her events in his childhood, jobs he had held, the service, his family, sports he liked, etc. He still, however, became involved in occasional altercations similar to those he had had frequently before. They usually occurred when he struck out at other patients who had accidentally bumped him. He felt that these acts were intentional, that other patients were testing him to see whether they could push him about. These incidents occurred with less and less frequency as the patient made conscious efforts to "stay out of trouble" so that eventually he would be allowed passes again with his mother,

Study 2. MR. V.[1]

First Hour of a Nurse-patient Relationship

The patient was lying on a bench on the porch adjacent to the dayroom of the admission unit. He sat up when the nurse was introduced to him. As he combed his hair, he made room on the bench for the nurse to sit beside him.

P–1. What do you want to talk about?

N–2. What would you like to talk about? [*Reflecting question back to the patient.*]

P–3. I don't know where I should start. Is this an autobiography or what? I'm completely in the dark—don't know what is coming off. Now I see what you are doing. You write everything down. Do you want my diagnosis? [*The patient is expressing a need to know what is expected of him.*]

N–4. Well, I'd like to hear anything you tell me. [*Giving a broad opening. Too broad at this time.*]

P–5. I was born at a very early age and that's when my trouble began. That's a joke; you can write that too.

P–6. Read it back. I want to see what it sounds like.

P–7. Wouldn't it be better with a dictaphone?

P–8. You have a nice handwriting. You know, I can take one look at this and tell you are a very competent woman.

[1] No summarization of the patient's history is included, since the nurse herself did not have this information until much later in the relationship. To read the history before seeing the patient or too early in the relationship tends to create prejudgments and thoughts channeled along certain lines; the nurse may then be less open-minded and less observant.

N–9. Why do you say that? [*Requesting an explanation. The patient has reversed roles. The conversation is focused on the nurse. The nurse might say, "It isn't necessary to flatter me," and then proceed to discuss her purpose in spending time with the patient.*]

P–10. I can tell by the way you write. Your words are spaced out nicely. Shows that you are lackadaisical when you write.

N–11. Would you like to talk about something else? [*Suggesting a change of topic but not explaining why or what the patient might talk about.*]

P–12. Are you married? [*The patient has focused on the nurse because he does not know what is expected of him.*]

N–13. Why do you ask? [*Requesting an explanation.*]

P–14. I ask all attractive females, to see if they are eligible or not.

N–15. Yes, I am. *Remember* I'm Mrs. R. [*Giving information. To say "remember" is to imply either disapproval with a warning for the future or "Don't you remember. . . ? I just told you." The word should be omitted.*]

P–16. I can't find anyone. I should have gotten married at a ripe old age of 17. Then everything would have been all right.

P–17. Do you think I'm flirting? Actually I flirt with all the nurses.

P–18. I know just what is going to happen. Whoever reads this is going to say I'm in the right place. [*The patient needs to be told the purpose of the nurse's taking notes and their subsequent utilization.*]

P–19. What do you think my diagnosis is, hmm?

P–20. So far all this proves is I'm an egotist. I think I'll try this. Write everything down and read it back and see how it sounds. [*The patient is attempting to hide his discomfort with humor and sarcasm. The nurse seems unsure as to how to proceed.*]

P–21. This is fun, you know.

N–22. I would like to come and talk with you once a week, if I may. [*Giving some information about her role but not discussing her purpose in coming.*]

P–23. I'm simply flattered to death. A pretty nurse to come talk to me. I'm a little baby; I love attention.

P–24. You might as well put my diagnosis down. I'm diagnosed schizophrenic, undifferentiated type. Save the doctor from looking into my clinical record.

N–25. Do you think you would like to have me talk to you every week? [*Requesting the patient's evaluation, but this is too soon to ask him to commit himself, especially when he does not have sufficient information.*]

P–26. Yeah, I think I would love it. It's nice to have someone to talk to who is in contact. [*The patient has assumed that the relationship is to be a social one.*]

P–27. Yeah, I think it would be nice. You would get to know me and I would get to know you. Gee, haven't I got terrible English. It just goes to show you, I have no education.

P–28. You know, I'm very good at this; I could talk all day long and say nothing. [*The patient is telling the nurse that he is not saying anything. Obviously he needs an explanation of the purpose of the relationship and his role. Then, the nurse can let the patient take the initiative. If the nurse can put herself in the patient's place at this moment, perhaps she can grasp how he feels.*]

N–29. Get attention? [*Suggesting a possible explanation. She might ask, "What purpose would this serve?"*]

P–30. I could never understand why I was never able to impress women.

P–31. Let's see, you must be about 35 years old. Gee, that works all the time. You just tell a woman she looks about five years younger than she is.

N–32. Could you tell me why you feel this way? [*Requesting an explanation.*]

P–33. No. I don't feel this way. I know it's true. I was listening to Joyce Brothers on TV and she states it.

P–34. Any particular subject you like to talk about?

N–35. Well, I like to talk about things that would make you feel better. [*Giving broad opening. Perhaps better stated, ". . . about things that make you feel uncomfortable." The patient does not know what will make him feel better.*]

P–36. Actually, I'm down in the dumps.

N–37. In the dumps? [*Restating.*]

P–38. What's your name again?

N–39. Mrs. R. [*Giving information.*]

N–40. Tell me more about your feelings. [*Exploring. Appropriately getting back to the topic under discussion.*]

P–41. My emotions—outwardly I'm very calm, but inwardly I'm all stopped up.

P–42. What do they call all these tests when you look at inkblots?

N–43. It is called the Rorschach test. [*Giving information.*]

P–44. That's how I know. I read the report on them. The doctor don't know, but I read my whole clinical record. I know more about myself than they do now.

P–45. I got all these doctors up a tree, except Dr. S. He knows me like a book. He talked to me one time for a half hour and that's all he needed.

P–46. Are you getting cold?

N–47. Yes.

P–48. You want to sit inside?

N–49. Yes, please.

(They went inside; the patient asked for a light and lit a cigarette.)

P–50. See what subject we are on now—feeling. When I was a small boy, I was not the least bit concerned about other people's feelings. I thought the world revolved about me.

P–51. When I was just a little kid in school, I used to think why be miserable when I can be a real stinker.

P–52. When I was about seven years old, I got real infatuated with girls. I used to go to parochial school and would always pick the best-looking girl in class and sit next to her. The girls sat on one side and the boys on the other. I never could get any of the girls interested in me. I was very unpopular with the girls. By the time I reached my early teens, I didn't have one single girl friend; when all the other fellows went out on dates, I didn't have any. I felt rejected and I attribute this to the fact that I know nothing about women.

Because women are much better at hiding their emotions, and you never know if they like you or not. You end up all confused. And then when I went in the army, the same thing. All the fellows would go out with the fast women and I would end up in the barracks. One time this came to the attention of my commanding officer, and he tried to get the fellows to show me a good time. It was a lost cause. It didn't work out. One guy even introduced me to his best girl friend.

P–53. That's been my trouble in the woman department, all my life. That's why I'm in a mental institution. I just kept deteriorating, and I feel all my life I had an inadequate personality and I was always completely incompatible.

P–54. Let's see, what else can we talk about? We are on the subject of feelings. I think that covers it.

N–55. I think this might be a good time to end our conversation. I'll come again next Thursday and we can continue our discussion. [*Suggesting termination of conversation. This seems rather abrupt. If a few minutes are saved for summarizing, the patient is not left with the impression that he has been "turned off" after expressing some of his innermost feelings.*]

P–56. Yeah, and then I'll have my other personality. [*This may have been just joking, but not necessarily.*]

N–57. Good-bye, Mr. V. Have a happy Easter. I'll see you next Thursday.

The nurse was most nondirective, allowing the patient to take the initiative. And in the latter half of the interview, the patient expressed many of his feelings about himself. But the first half, in which both the patient and the nurse were uncomfortable, might have gone more smoothly if the nurse had discussed her role, the purpose of the relationship, the patient's role, and the nurse's notes. Since the nurse did not explain these things, she will have to do it sooner or later, preferably as early as possible, clarifying and reinforcing her explanations in later meetings as needed.

Once these things are done, the nurse can follow the patient's lead. Summarizing at the end each time, even briefly, is also helpful.

In this first hour the nurse might say: "My name is Mrs. R. I'm a psychiatric nurse [or whatever is the appropriate description]. I'll be spending some time with you individually on a regular basis [be as specific as possible, e.g., every Monday, Wednesday, Thursday, and Friday from 10 to 11 A.M.].

"You may use this time in any way that will be of value to you—for example, discussing your problems, expressing your thoughts and feelings, describing experiences that make you uncomfortable—anything that will help me to know you better as a person and that will help us (you and me) to identify and explore your difficulties in relating to and living with others in a satisfying manner. Perhaps as, together, you and I come to look at your problems and explore them, their solution will be less difficult. Is this clear?

"Perhaps you can begin now by talking about whatever is of most concern to you."

Study 3. *MR. KARL C.*______

A Relationship with a Suicidal Patient

The patient, aged 42, was admitted to the hospital as a transfer in 1959. On admission he was well oriented but tense and agitated. His mood was described as one of depression and irritability. He readily admitted to suicidal and assaultive ideation. The patient was assigned to a unit providing maximum supervision. He continually inflicted slight burns on his arm with cigarettes, and between August and November, 1960, he made two attempts at burning his clothes. The latter attempt resulted in severe second- and third-degree burns of the chest and neck. The patient continued to express suicidal ideas and would bang his head against the wall, try to burn his hair, etc. Prior to the beginning of this nurse-patient relationship, he was described by the ward physician as "talking of suicide, but quiet, cooperative, and occupies himself well."

First Hour

N–1. Karl, I am going to spend some time each day with you. I will write down everything I say and, of course, your response. [*Giving information. Areas of information are not to be neglected, and it is important for the nurse to present her role.*]

P–2. Why don't you commit suicide?

N–3. I don't want to commit suicide. I like to live and I also have a child. [*Giving information. Informing the patient of facts builds up trust, gives greater knowledge for decisions or realistic conclusions.*]

P–4. Why don't you take him with you? You would be better off dead.

N–5. I don't like to talk about death or suicide; it's very morbid. [*Rejecting. Topic is rejected and closed from further exploration. Therapeutic interaction ceases.*]

Second Hour

N–1. Hello, Karl. [*Giving recognition. Greeting the patient gives recognition to him as a person. To use his surname, Mr. C., is preferable.*]

P–2. This is kinda silly, don't you think?

N–3. Don't you think we are trying to help you? [*Encouraging evaluation. The patient is asked to consider events and to evaluate the effects on him personally.*]

P–4. Don't be silly. I want to be dead, but they won't let me.

N–5. Why do you want to be dead? [*Requesting an explanation. The patient is asked to give reason for his thoughts before he is able to do so.*]

P–6. I lived with a girl. She committed suicide. I'm alone now.

N–7. With all these people around you, do you feel alone? [*Encouraging evaluation. The patient is asked to consider people and to evaluate their effects on him personally. The nurse should explore the patient's comment, "I'm alone now."*]

P–8. God wants me dead.

N–9. How do you know God wants you dead? [*Encouraging description of perceptions. Asking the patient to describe things as he sees them.*]

P–10. Over his heart in me.

N–11. Do you think God's heart is in you? [*Seeking clarification. Having a single idea mutually understood maintains communication.*]

P–12. No, on me.

N–13. What makes you think that? [*Indicating existence of external source.*]

P–14. I know so.

N–15. What would you like to do when you leave here? [*Introducing an unrelated topic. The initiative is taken from the patient. The nurse is now directing.*]

P–16. Commit suicide. My life is over. I would like somebody to leave the door open. I would jump off the water tower.

N–17. You lived in Germany; was it better there? [*Encouraging comparison. Comparing experiences brings out similar themes, and the patient becomes aware of a semblance of continuity in his life.*]

P–18. Look at these people who are kept here. What is outside for them? They are too old to enjoy life. I'm 41. God and my wife want me dead.

N–19. Did your wife tell you she wants you dead? [*Exploring. Patients* *sometimes deal only superficially to test the nurse's interest. The nurse looks further into the subject.*]

P–20. She threw me matches—other ways too, but it is personal.

N–21. Tell me about your happier days. [*Encouraging comparison.*]

P–22. That's past. It ended in 1950. I don't want to talk about it.

N–23. Tell me about your school days. [*Probing. The nurse is questioning and putting the patient on the defensive. He may feel that he has to answer the question.*]

P–24. I might have gotten further if it hadn't been for the operation in 1921—I was one year old.

N–25. I guess we had better call it quits for today. [*The nurse should indicate at the beginning of the period approximately how much time she will be spending with the patient. This will avoid abrupt endings such as this.*]

P–26. All right. Good-bye.

Third Hour

N–1. Hello, Karl.

P–2. I'd like a dog or cat.

N–3. What brought this to your mind? [*Exploring. The patient may be testing the nurse's interest. The nurse looks further into the subject.*]

P–4. I saw a cat today.

N–5. What did you think of the hula dancer? [*Introducing an unrelated topic. The initiative is taken from the patient. The nurse is now directing.*]

N–6. You tell me what you thought of her. [*Probing. The nurse is questioning and putting the patient on the defensive. He may feel that he has to answer the question.*]

P–7. She was good. This is kinda silly. Don't you think we are wasting time?

N–8. Whose time are we wasting? [*Seeking clarification. The patient knows when he is not understood and may stop communicating. His ideas must be mutually understood. Also, the meaning to the patient of "silly" should be explored. He has used it quite frequently—perhaps to imply "meaningless" or "hopeless."*]

P–9. I'm not worrying about my time; it's yours. I have no problems that death wouldn't solve. The only excuse for my continued existence would be massive suicide production among Americans. I know fully well I do not so produce. Therefore, death is the only answer both ways.

N–10. Couldn't we discuss something pleasant for a change? [*Rejecting. The patient's idea is ignored and/or minimized. He feels rejected, and interaction may cease.*]

P–11. Such as?

N–12. There are many things. Travel for one. [*Introducing an unrelated topic. The initiative is taken from the patient. The nurse is now directing.*]

N–13. Which country did you like the best? [*Encouraging evaluation. The patient is asked to consider events and to evaluate their effects on him personally.*]

P–14. India, because I almost had an accident that would have killed me.

N–15. Tell me about it? [*Exploring. Examining the subject more fully.*]

P–16. Airplane almost cracked up. If it had, I wouldn't be sitting in ______. What is the purpose of this? I suppose it's psychoanalytical.

N–17. No. I'm not qualified for that. I'm hoping my spending time with you will in some way help you. [*Giving information. The nurse is relating facts when asked a question. This develops trust and enhances the relationship. The nurse may have been less vague as to how it may be of value.*]

P–18. Whose problem do you think is more severe, mine or E.'s?

N–19. You both have problems, but they are so different, it would be hard to say. [*Giving information. The nurse by relating facts gives the patient information he may use in coming to more realistic conclusions.*]

N–20. Which do you think? [*Reflecting. The patient is requested to give an opinion on the topic of discussion. The nurse shows an interest in his views.*]

P–21. I think E.'s are.

N–22. Why do you think this? [*Requesting an explanation. The patient is asked to give reason for his thoughts before he is able to do so. Description and comparison might be encouraged.*]

P–23. He isn't suicidal—why wouldn't they be?

(Silence.)

N–24. Good night, Karl. [*The patient seems to imply that having a solution lessens his own problem. The nurse closes much too abruptly.*]

Fourth Hour

N–1. What's the good news today, Karl? [*The nurse has opened the conversation with a broad comment, but one not appropriate for a depressed patient.*]

P–2. No good news.

N–3. What about the book you have been reading? [*Introducing an unrelated topic. The initiative is taken from the patient. The nurse is now directing.*]

P–4. I read to kill time.

N–5. Don't you like to read? [*Disapproving. The nurse implies that the patient should like to read and would be considered unfavorably if he does not.*]

P–6. No. It's been years since I had any liquor. I have a taste for Chinese food.

N–7. Did you drink before you came here? [*Exploring. The nurse looks further into the subject.*]

P–8. Yes. It was my only pleasure in life. I'd like some Chinese food. Egg foo yung, sweet and sour pork.

N–9. Only one way to appease that appetite, Karl. Guess you know how. [*Testing. Appraising the patient's degree of insight by attempting to convince him of the extent of his incapacity.*]

P–10. No. How?

N–11. Well, I'm sure it will not be here. [*Testing.*]

P–12. Oh, you mean if I escape.

N–13. No, I don't mean that. [*Disagreeing. The nurse implies that the patient is wrong. He must then defend his position by strengthening his ideas.*]

P–14. I would have no place to go. No one wants me. You have two pages; don't you think that's enough?

N–15. All right, Karl, we will call it a day until tomorrow. [*Rejecting. The nurse fails to explore the patient's expressed topic and therapeutic interaction ceases.*]

Suicidal patients often ask to be rejected. Unknowingly, the nurse rejected him twice at the close of this discussion: (1) The patient said, "No one wants me." By not following up on this comment in any way, the nurse implied that it was true. (2) The patient said, "Don't you think that's enough?" By agreeing, the nurse implied that she had had enough. It goes without saying that the nurse did not intend to give this impression, but does the patient know this? By letting the patient think otherwise, the nurse let him prove to himself how right he is about life's not being worth living.

Fifth Hour

N–1. Come on, Karl, let's have a little conversation. [*Offering broad opening, but in a demanding manner.*]

P–2. I'm interested in sleep, especially permanent sleep.

N–3. I told you I don't want to discuss suicide. [*Rejecting. The nurse fails to explore the patient's expressed topic, and therapeutic interaction may cease.*]

P–4. That's all that is on my mind.

N–5. Why can't an intelligent man such as you think of something else? [*Disapproving. The nurse passes judgment on the patient's thoughts and actions.*]

P–6. There is nothing else for me.

N–7. Why? [*Requesting an explanation. The patient is asked to give reasons for his thoughts before he is able to do so.*]

P–8. My life ended some time ago.

N–9. Why? [*Requesting an explanation. The patient is again asked to give reason for his thoughts before he is able to do so.*]

P–10. Someone died—who may or may not have been my wife.

N–11. I thought your wife was living. [*Seeking clarification. Having a single idea mutually understood maintains communication.*]

P–12. I don't think so. I asked her to commit suicide; she may or may not have.

N–13. There's that word again. [*Rejecting. The nurse fails to explore the patient's expressed topic, and therapeutic interaction may cease.*]

P–14. That's all that is on my mind. Let's call it quits. I'm sleepy. Could you stand this place 14 hours a day?

N–15. If you don't like it here, why don't you help us to help you? First, by putting thoughts of suicide from your mind. [*Advising. Indicating to the patient that he is unable to direct himself.*]

P–16. With all these patients wanting your help, why do you waste it on me?

N–17. I don't think I'm wasting my time. [*Offering self. Expressing her desire to be of help and her faith in his potential for growth.*]

P–18. (Looking at television.) I don't like Westerns. They are addressed to a two-and-a-half-year-old.

N–19. What do you like? [*Exploring. Examining a subject more fully* *to establish the feeling that the nurse is interested in the patient's experiences.*]

P–20. Death—my friend.

N–21. Good-bye, Karl. [*Abrupt closing and departure.*]

The nurse continues to reject the topic of suicide as she feels that it is not "good" for the patient to think about it. By exploring the topic, the nurse may better understand what the patient's needs are. Very little is known, up to this point, about why the patient wants to die and also what he has to live for. Finding a reason for living makes suicide unnecessary. Without satisfying human relationships, such reason is not likely to be found.

Sixth Hour

N–1. Hello, Karl.

P–2. (Watching a movie.) It's called, "The Trapp Family." I would have liked to have raised five children.

N–3. Do you have any? [*Exploring. The patient may be testing the nurse's interest. The nurse looks further into the subject.*]

P–4. No.

N–5. Does this bring back pleasant memories of when you were a young child? [*Exploring. The nurse continues to examine the subject to demonstrate her interest in the patient.*]

P–6. No. I always wanted to be dead.

N–7. I can't imagine this being so at the age of five or six. [*Voicing doubt. The patient becomes aware that the nurse finds this hard to believe. The patient is then encouraged to re-evaluate what has been said.*]

P–8. These are the unfortunate facts. All my life I have been frustrated. What do you think of this movie?

N–9. I like it very much. Don't you? [*Making stereotyped comments. Patterned replies lack therapeutic value in a nurse-patient relationship.*]

P–10. Put down "So do I" and let's call it a day.

N–11. I must go, Karl. You can tell me how this ends tomorrow. [*The nurse expresses more interest in the movie than in the patient. Movie time is certainly not a desirable time for establishing verbal communication.*]

The nurse needs to know what does have meaning for the patient. Evidently hospital life is of no value to him and appears to be an added burden. The nurse must learn how it can be more meaningful. What are the patient's needs? Can the nurse meet any? How? What are his interests? If it is true that "all my life I have been frustrated," what is it the patient has wanted out of life and never had? What has he wanted to do? The nurse may ask him to describe the kind of life he would enjoy living if he could have it just as he wishes.

Seventh Hour

N–1. Seems like a long time since our last chat. [*Making an observation. The nurse offers the patient something to which he may respond when ready.*]

P–2. Yep. You wanted me to remember the last of the movie.

N–3. Okay, tell me. [*Offering a general lead. Encouraging the patient to direct the conversation and assuring him of the nurse's interest.*]

P–4. Germans take over Austria. They escape to—of all places—New York. At first they have financial difficulties, but later they support themselves by singing. They buy themselves a house on Long Island. Presumably, they live happily ever after.

(The ward physician stopped and spoke to the patient. He told the physician she should commit suicide and take her children with her. The nurse and the doctor told the patient that life was worth living and beautiful.)

P–5. Purpose of the human species is the massive minimization of hell for all living, not for life to be beautiful for the few years of youth.

N–6. My mother used to say to us: "Laugh and the world laughs with you. Cry and you cry alone." Do you believe this? [*Making stereotyped comments. Patterned replies lack therapeutic value in a nurse-patient relationship.*]

P–7. Your mother had to tell you that. If she didn't, she would lose her children, and she was afraid she might get hurt.

N–8. I hardly agree with you on that. I think it is true. [*Disagreeing. The nurse is implying that the patient is wrong. He must then defend his position by strengthening his ideas.*]

P–9. The good Lord in heaven is praying for suicides among Americans. So am I.

N–10. Why Americans? [*Seeking clarification. The nurse, by seeking to have a single idea mutually understood, maintains communication.*]

P–11. Because they sit on top of something horrifying.

N–12. What could that be? [*Encouraging description of perceptions. Asking the patient to describe things as he sees them. Exploring. The nurse delves further.*]

P–13. In the face of unduly long periods in hell, only the straightest type of thinking can be permitted. Why don't Americans lay down and die?

N–14. Do you think life would have been different for you if you hadn't come to America? [*Encouraging comparison. The nurse, by comparing experiences, brings out differences and helps the patient evaluate the influence of events and persons on his life.*]

P–15. I should have been put out at birth. There would have been no life. I was raised for that purpose. I would have killed myself as a small child. Unfortunately, my head was never my own.

N–16. I thought today would be far more pleasant as far as our conversation. I am not (as you know) a morbid person. [*Disapproving. The nurse implies that the patient is expected to please her. Rejecting. The topic of conversation is closed off from further exploration. The nurse should have considered whether the patient felt someone did his thinking for him. Who? What kind of decisions were made for him?*]

P–17. I've had enough for one day.

N–18. All right, we will watch the movies. [*The nurse may find it helpful to find out in greater detail in what ways life is so burdensome.*]

Eighth Hour

N–1. Let's have a gay, pleasant conversation today. No suicide or death, please. [*Using denial. The nurse's comment prevents discussion of a problem that she may have qualms about. Further exploration of the patient's problems is closed off. Rejecting. Refusing to discuss the patient's expressed feelings.*]

P–2. Do unto others as you would all others do unto you.

N–3. Why do you think that particular saying goes at this time? [*Requesting an explanation.*]

P–4. It goes at any time.

N–5. True. [*Agreeing. The nurse indicates her accord with the patient; however, it leaves him with less opportunity to later modify his point of view.*]

N–6. Tell me about the different sports you enjoyed as a boy. [*Introducing an unrelated topic. The nurse has changed the topic of conversation and has taken the initiative.*]

P–7. Soccer, Ping-pong, tennis, ice skating, athletics, swimming, dancing, skiing.

N–8. You did all these things? [*Exploring. The nurse assures the patient of her interest by examining the patient's experiences.*]

P–9. I am actually two people, and I never know which one the questions are addressed to.

N–10. What makes you think you are two people? [*Indicating existence of external source. The nurse implies that outside influences make him feel this way. The patient may have been asked to describe the "two people."*]

P–11. I know so.

N–12. Do you hear voices? [*Introducing an unrelated topic. The nurse has changed the topic of conversation and has taken the initiative. She might say, "Tell me about this."*]

P–13. What's the difference between this place and animals in a zoo? Answer that.

N–14. Animals can't talk, eat with silver, enjoy ward parties, movies, visitors, and so forth. [*Giving literal response. The patient is expressing feeling, and the nurse indicates her inability to understand the feelings expressed by dealing factually with the comment.*]

P–15. I can't answer that properly without mentioning suicide.

N–16. Why? [*Requesting an explanation. Asking the patient to give reasons for his feelings before he has learned to understand them himself.*]

P–17. If the mental patient had any mentality, they would commit suicide.

N–18. I disagree with you. I know many patients who recovered and are now living a normal happy life. [*Disagreeing. The nurse implies that the patient is wrong. He must defend his position by strengthening his ideas. Reassuring. The attempt to relieve the patient's anxiety by minimizing the existing situation only increases his feeling of not being understood. He is not "many patients."*]

P–19. If they loved their wives, they would help her get rid of a cripple whether they asked them or not.

N–20. Most wives love their husbands and do not want to get rid of them, especially when they are sick. [*Reassuring. Attempting to relieve the patient's anxiety by minimizing the comment expressed only increases his feeling of being misunderstood.*]

P–21. Why don't they just kill themselves and give their wives a chance for a second husband whom they would love just as much and who have not as yet given evidence in the direction of a tendency to become disabled cripples?

N–22. I'm sure the wives of these patients would not agree with you. [*Disagreeing. The nurse has implied that the patient is wrong. He must defend his position by strengthening his ideas. It should be considered whether the patient is expressing concern about his wife and her feelings.*]

P–23. I'm sure they would agree with me, but they wouldn't admit it. As long as they can cling to the first husband, they haven't a chance to look for the second one. The prospect of having two might not be a pleasant one. That is no excuse for the husband to take advantage of her fears and fail to give her a second chance.

N–24. Somehow we always end on this tone when it should be a more pleasant one, don't you think? [*Disapproving. The nurse has placed a judgmental value on the patient's comment. It must be understood that these meetings do not have to be "pleasant." The nurse strives toward the goal of developing a productive relationship. To do so, she must allow free expression of the patient's thoughts and feelings.*]

P–25. We are no longer children, and a pleasant life is reserved for the young. For adults, life is earnest and grim. You are referred back to yesterday's discussion. Enough is enough. Let's quit.

N–26. All right, Karl. I will see you tomorrow. [*Complying. Giving information.*]

The patient's description of adult life in this past meeting as being "earnest and grim" is much less negative than anything he has expressed about it thus far. These are the most realistic words he has used, since life is not all sweetness and light; it is earnest and often grim.

Ninth Hour

N–1. Hello, Karl. I haven't seen you for awhile. I have been off for a few days. [*Giving recognition. Greeting the patient gives recognition to him as a person. Giving information.*]

P–2. Where were you? Were you sick?

N–3. No, I had emergency annual leave for personal reasons. [*Giving information. Answering the patient's questions factually builds up trust and gives him a greater body of knowledge.*]

P–4. I would like to be dead. Therefore, I am frustrated.

N–5. Describe this feeling to me. [*Encouraging description of perception. Asking the patient to describe his feelings as he perceives them. Most appropriate.*]

P–6. From the time I get up in the morning till the time I lay down to sleep at night, all I can think of is how nice it would be to be dead, and yet I am still deprived of the right to take my own life. Incidentally, a zoo is more humane than this institution. No one ever bothers zoo animals, and they are safe from attack or physical manhandling of any type. No one ever feels safe in here.

N–7. Do you feel you are being bothered and manhandled here? [*Reflecting. The nurse is requesting the patient to express an opinion and shows an interest in his views.*]

P–8. No one ever feels safe here.

N–9. In what way do you feel that you are not safe? [*Encouraging description of perceptions. Encouraging the patient to describe his perceptions as he sees them. Much more useful than "defending" the hospital.*]

P–10. They want me to make my bed in the morning in spite of the fact I'm an involuntary patient and am being kept alive against my will.

N–11. Most patients make their beds. [*Giving information. Answering the patient's questions factually builds up trust and gives him a greater body of knowledge.*]

P–12. They are voluntary patients.

N–13. How long have you had this desire to commit suicide? [*Attempting to place in sequence. Placing events in their proper sequence enables the nurse and the patient to see them as they relate to each other and the whole. Better expressed in his words, "to cease to be alive?"*]

P–14. Since 1953. I have never changed my mind.

N–15. What happened then to take your desire to live away? [*Encouraging description of perceptions. Encouraging the patient to describe his perceptions as he sees them.*]

P–16. Attendants in a mental institution beat me up and injured my liver, took away my sense of physical safety, plus the fact I had enough of the operation and of being used.

N–17. Who do you feel was using you? [*Seeking clarification. Having a single idea mutually understood enhances the continuation of communication between the nurse and the patient.*]

P–18. What sits on top of America and the American people?

N–19. What sits on top of America? [*Restating. Repeating what the patient has said in almost the same words. Seeking clarification. Having a single idea mutually understood maintains communication.*]

P–20. How should I know? You tell me. Something does.

N–21. I never knew that something sat on top of America. Tell me about it. [*Exploring. The patient is testing the nurse's interest by dealing *superficially. The nurse must examine further. Encouraging description of perceptions. Encouraging the patient to describe his perceptions as he sees them.*]

P–22. No comment.

N–23. That doesn't tell me much, does it? [*Making an observation.*]

P–24. If you don't know, you wouldn't want to know.

N–25. I must want to know or I wouldn't be asking you. [*Offering self. Presenting oneself unconditionally in order that the patient feels free to make himself understood.*]

P–26. Don't you think the personnel have too much power over the mental patient?

N–27. We only want to help you, hoping some day you will want to live and enjoy life again. [*Giving information. Presenting facts when the patient indicates a need for information.*]

P–28. Why don't you admit that you know better?

N–29. It is the purpose of the nurses and the doctors to save lives, not to take them. Surely you know this. [*Giving information. Presenting facts when the patient indicates a need for information. The nurse should avoid sounding as though she is defending herself. This only puts her in opposition to the patient.*]

P–30. Let's quit for the day.

N–31. All right.

The nurse attempts to defend the personnel, but this will not change his feelings about them. It will also put the patient in opposition to her. The nurse should try to understand what led him to feel this way—this does not mean that she must agree. The patient's past difficult experiences in life are worth exploring. The nurse should encourage the patient to discuss whatever experiences he feels would help her understand him better as a person.

Tenth Hour

N–1. Karl, do you remember what first caused your depressed feelings? [*Requesting an explanation. Perhaps better worded, "Tell me what happened at the time you first felt depressed."*]

P–2. I can't answer that. I suggest the patients in _____ be put out.

N–3. Out where? [*Seeking clarification. Having a single idea mutually understood enhances the continuation of communication.*]

P–4. Out of life. They would be better off dead. Those are the facts. This whole thing is silly.

N–5. You think so, but are you enjoying it? [*Encouraging evaluation. The patient is asked to consider this experience and to evaluate the effects on him personally. The nurse might have asked, "Does this make you feel uncomfortable?"*]

P–6. We can never understand each other, for I am guided by fear of God, and living Americans, except for me, have no religion.

N–7. I have a religion, and I am guided by fear of God. [*Disagreeing. Implying that the patient is wrong. He must defend his position by strengthening his ideas. The nurse appears to be defending herself rather than trying to understand what the patient means.*]

P–8. If it were true, you would commit suicide.

N–9. You feel that those who are guided by God should commit suicide. [*Restating. Repeating what the patient has said in almost the same words gives evidence to him that an idea has been communicated effectively.*]

P–10. I know so.

N–11. How do you know this? [*Encouraging description of perceptions. Encouraging the patient to describe his ideas as he sees them. Better worded, "What happened to give you this impression?"*]

P–12. God cares about helping the worst off amongst all living on this planet. The only way they can be helped is if Americans commit suicide. Therefore, God wants Americans to commit suicide. While there is no God, people ought to proceed on the assumption that there was and guide themselves accordingly. Why aren't you dead? What we need in this world is more good books.

N–13. Do you like to read? And what do you like to read? [*Exploring. Examining a subject more fully to establish the feeling of the nurse's interest in the patient's habits. However, the patient has changed the subject without the nurse's trying to understand what he has been saying.*]

P–14. Yes. Short stories. When will I be able to die? Would you let me die if I set myself on fire?

N–15. I think I should take one question at a time. Describe to me this feeling you must have to want to die so badly. [*Encouraging description of perceptions. Encouraging the patient to describe his feelings.*]

P–16. Give me liberty or give me death. If I had my liberty, I would kill myself.

N–17. That is more of a statement than explaining a feeling. [*Encouraging description of perceptions. Encouraging the patient to describe his feelings as he perceives them. Better worded, "than describing a feeling."*]

P–18. They used big words to defend slavery. Suicide is supposed to be a defense against unjust abuse of the helpless.

N–19. You feel helpless? [*Attempting to translate into feeling. The nurse recognizes the patient's comment as expressing his feelings and has attempted to verbalize them.*]

P–20. Certainly. I am merely a body pushed through each day by means of physical threats. "Is life so sweet or peace so dear as to be purchased with price of chains of slavery?" The operation of a mental institution is therefore an unAmerican activity. The patients ought to be put out. Mental institutions are in violation of the spirit of the founders of the republic.

N–21. Have you a plan for the people who are sick? [*Exploring. Examining a subject more fully to establish the feeling of the nurse's interest in the patient's idea.*]

(No response.)

The nurse learned a great deal about the patient's feelings. Living for a long period in a hospital on a locked ward is far from conducive to feelings of hope and satisfaction. The nurse needs to find ways of making his present life more satisfying.

The nurse also needs to know more about his delusional ideas. The patient gives the impression that he feels he must die to help others and that Americans are somehow the cause of all the misery in the rest of the world. It may be that the patient feels that Americans have so much and others so little because we are depriving others, and if Americans die, others will live better.

The nurse should try to determine exactly what the patient does mean and how the suicide of Americans will save the world. Then, perhaps, the nurse can ask if there are any alternatives or other courses of action for Americans who want to help others.

The nurse is getting the patient to express himself more fully and to describe his feelings and points of view. The nurse is apparently beginning to understand the patient's feelings. This tends to raise the patient's self-esteem and make life more satisfying.

Eleventh Hour

N–1. Good afternoon, Karl. [*Giving recognition. Greeting the patient by name gives recognition to him as a person.*]

P–2. What happened to Dr. B.? I haven't seen her.

N–3. I understand she has the flu, along with a good many others. [*Giving information. Presenting facts when the patient indicates a need for information.*]

P–4. I had the flu.

N–5. Since you have been in this hospital? [*Attempting to place in sequence. This enables the nurse and the patient to place events in their proper place as they relate to other events.*]

P–6. No. I don't remember where. Look, I'm so sleepy; how can you have the heart to wake me?

N–7. If you sleep all day, how can you sleep at night? [*Exploring. Delving into the topic.*]

P–8. I don't. I lay awake thinking.

N–9. Tell me about it. [*Exploring. Examining the subject more fully.*]

P–10. Nothing to tell. Today isn't our day. If you would all die, I could sleep forever. Tell me about your husband.

N–11. What would you like to know? [*Seeking clarification. Having a single idea mutually understood enhances the continuation of communications. However, it would have been better for the nurse to indicate that the time should be spent talking about him.*]

P–12. Whatever is worth knowing.

N–13. He is tall, handsome, and has a terrific sense of humor. [*Giving information. Presenting facts when the patient indicates a need for information. However, this is information of a personal nature and of little therapeutic value.*]

P–14. Am I giving you an inferiority complex?

N–15. No, Karl, I'm not getting a complex. Do you think I should? [*Disagreeing. The nurse has implied that the patient is wrong. He must defend his position by strengthening his ideas. Reflecting. Directing the question back to the patient.*]

P–16. I can't think of anything today.

N–17. All right, maybe we will have a better time tomorrow. Many days I don't feel much like talking either. I will see you tomorrow. [*Accepting. The nurse is again being nonjudgmental but indicates to the patient that she has heard and follows the comment made. The nurse should emphasize the fact that the patient does not have to talk all the time she is there.*]

The patient needs to know that the nurse is not just interested in him when he is having a good day. Patients who are depressed tend to feel that others have little real interest in them and think only of themselves. Slighting the patient in the smallest manner may be interpreted as demonstrating his lack of worth. Leaving the patient when he is not contributing to the discussion and talking about herself are instances when the nurse may give this impression.

The nurse must make every attempt to demonstrate to such a patient that she is genuinely interested in his welfare,

Twelfth Hour

N–1. Hello, Karl. This has been an exciting day, hasn't it? [This was the day of astronaut John Glenn's voyage into space.] [*Giving recognition. Greeting the patient by name gives recognition to him as a person.*]

P–2. I wish I was the astronaut. I would escape from the human species.

N–3. You feel the need for escape? [*Reflecting. Directing the feeling expressed back to the patient.*]

P–4. Yes, because the human species won't let me die.

N–5. What could possibly have happened to you to make you feel this way? [*Encouraging description of perceptions. Encouraging the patient to describe his feelings as he sees them.*]

P–6. I lost my wife. Also, when I was eighteen years old, I loved a girl, and since I couldn't marry her, I should have committed suicide. They wouldn't let me.

N–7. Tell me about this girl. [*Exploring. Examining the subject more fully.*]

P–8. Her name was Kathy, and all of Chicago knew us. They knew us before we came to Chicago. I met her in Vienna. I found out she lived in Chicago, so I went there. I get in trouble, and no one would speak to me. But they wouldn't let me die. I couldn't marry her because I didn't have the means to support her.

N–9. Do you know what happened to her? [*Exploring.*]

P–10. No.

N–11. What kind of trouble did you get in? [*Exploring. The nurse pursues the subject and attempts to demonstrate her interest in the patient's experiences.*]

P–12. This is not confessing.

N–13. Of course not. There isn't any reason for you to confess to me. So you tell me about the wife you said you lost. She wasn't Kathy was she? [*Exploring. Examining the subject more fully to establish the feeling of the nurse's interest in the patient's experience. It is important to note that the nurse continued to refer to the subject in discussion and did not change the topic.*]

P–14. No. Her name was Mary. I won't talk about her—she wants me dead.

This was an abrupt ending. The nurse might have said, "This earlier experience must have been a very unhappy one for you. It would seem that it relates to your present feelings. Perhaps you can discuss it further with me tomorrow."

Thirteenth Hour

N–1. Good afternoon, Karl. [*Giving recognition. Greeting the patient by name gives recognition to him as a person.*]

P–2. Good afternoon. I have told you everything I have to tell. Do you know what it feels like to drag a dead body through a day, with no end in sight?

N–3. Describe this feeling to me. [*Encouraging description of perception. Encouraging the patient to describe his feelings as he sees them.*]

P–4. I hate everyone. Why won't they let me die?

N–5. What caused you to have this feeling of wanting to die? [*Requesting an explanation. Asking the patient to give reasons for his feelings before he has learned to understand them himself.*]

P–6. I have always had it. I am an orphan. There is no love ever.

N–7. Aren't your mother and father living? [*Testing. Appraising the patient's degree of insight by attempting to convince him of the extent of his incapacity. The nurse might have said, "You feel that you don't know your parents?"*]

P–8. I was kidnapped at birth from my mother and father and never met them.

N–9. Tell me about your sister. [*Introducing an unrelated topic. The nurse has changed the topic of conversation and has taken the initiative. She could say, "I don't follow you. Tell me more about this."*]

P–10. I have no sister, that I ever met. I have one that played the part.

N–11. Did she play it well? [*Giving a literal response. The patient is expressing feeling, and the nurse indicates her inability to follow the thought. The nurse implies that she was playing the part. A more appropriate response might have been, "She seemed to be playing a part."*]

P–12. Yes, they were all good actors. When are you going to let me die? That's all this is—dragging dead bodies through the day. Answer this question for me. Are they going to let me die?

N–13. We don't want any of our patients to die. We want to see them and you get well. [*Giving information. Presenting facts when the patient indicates a need for information.*]

P–14. You are a good liar. I am not a patient. I am an involuntary prisoner.

N–15. I know you must feel like a prisoner; perhaps you could describe this feeling more in detail. [*Accepting. The nurse is being nonjudgmental but indicates to the patient that she has heard and follows the comment made. Encouraging description of perception. Asking the patient to supply more details.*]

P–16. The only liberty we have is that of selecting which unoccupied chair we choose to sit in. Also, we can walk back and forth on the floor of the dayroom. I would rather be dead. How long does it take to be a nurse?

N–17. It takes three years. [*Giving information. Presenting facts when the patient indicates a need for information.*]

P–18. It takes six years to be a doctor.

N–19. Would you like to be a doctor? [*Reflecting. Directing the topic to the patient personally.*]

P–20. No. Lack of personal integrity and absence of backbone is one of the factors.

N–21. I would like to understand this low opinion you have of yourself. [*Encouraging description of perception. Encouraging the patient to describe his feelings as he sees them. Attempting to translate into feeling. The nurse is attempting to understand how the patient must feel in order to express himself as he did.*]

The nurse should indicate to the patient that she cares for his welfare and comfort. In doing so, she should try to express herself in such a manner that the patient cannot twist its meaning to one of personal gain for the nurse.

The patient appears to give the impression that everyone is insincere by his comments that the nurse is a "liar" and that his sister "played a part." These feelings should be explored further in an attempt to uncover their origin. He seems to be saying that there was no sincere expression of love in his family.

Fourteenth Hour

N–1. Hello, Karl.

P–2. (Watching a movie.) All that whisky and I can't get any.

N–3. Were you a drinker in your day? [*Exploring. Examining the subject more fully.*]

P–4. Yes. I enjoyed drinking. Occasionally I would get drunk.

N–5. Did drinking make you feel gay or depressed? [*Encouraging evaluation. The patient is asked to consider events and to evaluate their effects on him.*]

P–6. Gay.

N–7. Did you enjoy your visitor yesterday? Tell me about it. [*Introducing an unrelated topic. The nurse has changed the topic of conversation and taken the initiative.*]

P–8. She isn't my sister. I asked her about a method to commit suicide and she refused. That was all.

N–9. Is she married? [*Probing. Asking unwarranted questions. The patient does not seem to welcome pursuit of this subject. In addition, the nurse ceases to focus on the patient.*]

P–10. Yes. She has one child, 28 years old. A boy. He isn't married.

N–11. She must be older than you. [*Probing.*]

P–12. Yes, by nine years.

N–13. Did she come to this country with you? [*Probing.*]

P–14. No. She came before me, about a year. In 1937. I want to be dead so badly I can taste it.

N–15. What a terrible feeling that must be. [*Accepting. The nurse is being nonjudgmental but indicates to the patient that she has heard and follows the comment made.*]

P–16. It is terrible, especially when there is no hope of dying. You all watch me too closely.

N–17. We are trying to help you, trying to understand. [*Offering self. Presenting oneself unconditionally in order that the patient feels free to make himself understood.*]

This relationship was then interrupted for a period of time while the nurse was on night duty in other areas of the hospital. If the patient was prepared for this interruption, the interaction notes do not indicate this.

Study 4. *MR. W. B.*

Excerpts from a Nurse-patient Relationship

The patient, aged 36, is the second of six surviving children of a total of 11. The home broke up when the patient was a child of five and was in the hospital for a herniorrhaphy. He was taken by the aid society and then placed with his sister and three brothers in a foster home. Periods of several months were spent with four different families. At the age of 10 the boy was sent to a residential school and following this a reformatory. While at the latter, he was told that his mother had died. He was then 17. A series of odd jobs followed, after which he was accepted by the Army. He spent two years of World War II in the European theater, taking part in the air offensive of the Normandy invasion. In 1949 he was admitted to a state hospital. After a stay of seven and a half years, he was transferred to a Veterans Administration hospital. A few days before the nurse-patient relationship began, his doctor described the patient as "regressed, withdrawn, confused, untidy, and disoriented."

First Hour

N–1. Is there something you'd like to talk about? [*Giving a broad opening comment.*]

P–2. Anything. What would you like to talk about?

N–3. Shall we talk about you? [*Tentatively suggesting a general topic.*]

P–4. What about?

N–5. Oh, about how you feel. [*Suggesting topic. Better worded, ". . . about your feelings."*]

P–6. Well, concerning the facts, it's mighty serious, whichever way it goes. I'm beginning to like the words. It makes me—uh—over across the riverside—the fact where it went was the stovepipe—it was 25 to 50 roads.

N–7. Twenty-five to fifty roads? [*Restating.*]

P–8. To which it would be a fact where it would go at. . . .

N–9. I don't think I understand. [*Seeking clarification. Better stated, "I don't think I follow you."*]

P–10. Friday night—it was going over across the roadside—Thursday night it rained. It down where the fact it was going, wherever it got it was going down somewhere.

N–11. What is this you're talking about? [*Seeking clarification. Encouraging description.*]

P–12. A roadside dance where they're going. I was up there some place and I went down—there was a roadside over there—and they were doing things.

N–13. They were doing things. [*Restating.*]

P–14. In a way.

N–15. What kind of things? [*Exploring.*]

P–16. A little bit of manula—up and down where they were going—Friday night they were doing things.

Second Hour

N–1. What shall we talk about today? [*Giving a broad opening comment.*]

P–2. Oh, roses are red and violets are blue, I had a sweet little girl and she loved you. And then Friday night came around, and they was up and down by the place over there and away they went all over the place. It happened to be more than somebody would know. They happened to be —uh—it was more than most people would recognize. They went across the road. It was pretty far away. It happened to be pretty deep.

N–3. Pretty deep? [*Restating.*]

P–4. That Friday night it was. They got up there across the road—the way they were doing.

N–5. I don't understand what they were doing. [*Seeking clarification. The nurse might encourage description, "What is it they were doing?"*]

P–6. They were building an airplane. They happened to have different kinds of so-called zepladiols.

N–7. Zepladiols? [*Restating.*]

P–8. Yeah.

N–9. What is a zepladiol? [*Seeking clarification.*]

P–10. A partuly with a ziklifier.

N–11. What language is that? [*Exploring.*]

P–12. Hookamuka.

N–13. Did you make these words up? [*Exploring. Perhaps less threatening if worded, "Are these your own words?"*]

P–14. No, they're Spanish–Latin American.

N–15. I can't understand that. I'm trying to understand you. [*Seeking clarification. Offering self. The nurse might say, "These words have no meaning for me" or "What is it you're trying to tell me?"*]

Fourth Hour

P–1. These people think they're so smart and all. Sons of _____. Bastards.

N–2. These people make you angry? [*Reflecting.*]

P–3. They're no good. Never was no good.

N–4. What do they do that's making you angry? [*Encouraging description of perceptions.*]

P–5. I don't know—up by the road and aways they went. . . .

Sixth Hour

P–1. Friday night I was over by the place—I put down a place over yonder where it was going—a place where was a sadding sad—S-A-D. . . .

N–2. I know what "sad" is. [*Accepting.*]

P–3. Ever get sad, ever get lonely?

N–4. Yes. Were you sad? [*Reflecting.*]

P–5. No, I was move—uh—I never should have left Morristown. I was in a crowd that knew one another.

N–6. You lived in the town of Morristown? [*Exploring.*]

P–7. Years ago. He had a lot of friends.

N–8. Who? [*Seeking clarification.*]

P–9. Guy by the name of B. You can't understand why nobody comes to see you.

N–10. You were in the hospital then? [*Seeking clarification.*]

P–11. Yeah. I was in the hospital—seven years, say eight years. Some day—you stop and think—you're far away from your girl friend—you are far away, you know—up by the road, you think I might not have to do it, I'll never see her again you say—I don't know why I did it, I never give it a thought. (Started singing.)

N–12. You said you didn't know why you did it? [*Restating.*]

P–13. Oh, yeah, building airplanes. (Sang again.)

Tenth Hour

P–1. There ain't nothing exciting to do—like flying an airplane or racing down the road in a fast car. People don't want people around who are mentally sick. I got sick over in Germany—it was the Army's fault.

N–2. The Army's fault? [*Restating.*]

P–3. Starvation and drink. If they ain't going to give you nothing to eat—nothing you like. I got sick twice—in France and in Germany. In France it was my fault; I was drinking. In Belgium I got well again in three weeks' time. I was sick coming home—thinking I was a big-shot hero—I was no hero. I was afraid I was going to kill somebody. I didn't know nothing about spiritual things at that time.

N–4. What do you mean "spiritual things"? [*Seeking clarification and consensual validation. Better stated, "Tell me about the spiritual things."*]

P–5. It seemed like there was two of us. One of us was having a good time with a girl. I seen her in spiritual form on my cot.

N–6. Let's go back a minute and see if I've got this right. [*Reviewing.*]

P–7. What good's that going to do?

N–8. I want to understand. [*Offering self. Better worded, "I want to make certain that I'm following what you say."*]

(They went back over the notes.)

P–9. Maybe trying to think of myself as a hero was a way of trying to overcome my sickness—and it made it worse. I do that here sometimes, try to overcome one form of sickness with another.

Study 5. *MR. FRANK D.* ______

Excerpts from a Nurse-patient Relationship

The patient, aged 40, is one of 13 children. A sister committed suicide. At 16 he quit school in the eighth grade to assist with the farm work at home. In 1941 he was drafted into the Army. He spent time in Alaska and in the Aleutians with three months in combat. He was discharged on points in 1945. After a difficult time adjusting at home, he re-enlisted to get away from discord in the family. Sent to Germany, he was first hospitalized there about a year later. After six months in an Army hospital in the United States, he was transferred to a Veterans Administration hospital, where he has spent the last nine years. About two years after admission, he struck a patient with a barbell in the gymnasium. The patient died. Three months later, Mr. D. underwent a prefrontal lobotomy. He was considered to have shown only slight temporary improvement as a result of the operation. He has been on observation status continually since that time as a precaution against both homicide and suicide.

First Hour

P–1. I don't know what to talk about. I'd like to get transferred.

N–2. Transferred? [*Restating.*]

P–3. I'd like to get a privilege pass or a privilege card.

N–4. Some of the patients in this ward have privilege cards. [*Giving information.*]

P–5. In this building?

N–6. Yes. [*Repeating.*]

P–7. I'd like to go to the canteen. I don't want to hurt myself.

N–8. Hurt yourself? [*Restating.*]

P–9. I don't want to hurt myself. I sleep at night. I don't know anything about television. I don't have no visitors—nobody comes to see me.

N–10. I guess that must make it pretty lonely. [*Attempting to translate into feelings.*]

P–11. I don't want to talk about shock. I don't know anything about it.

N–12. You can talk about anything you want to. [*Giving a broad opening comment.*]

P–13. I don't know anything about black.

N–14. Black? [*Restating.*]

P–15. Black.

N–16. What do you mean? [*Seeking clarification. Better worded, "What idea are you using this word to convey?"*]

P–17. I see it in the morning. I think I see it in the morning when I drink water.

N–18. You see "black" when you drink water? [*Restating.*]

P–19. No. I like to eat fruit.

N–20. Where does this "black" come in? [*Seeking clarification.*]

P–21. That's what I don't know.

N–22. What does it look like when you see "black"? [*Encouraging description of perceptions.*]

P–23. They're horses—I think they're farm horses. I've seen them in coal mines.

N–24. Farm horses in coal mines? [*Restating.*]

P–25. I've seen them in coal mines.

Third Hour

P–1. I wish I'd got away with a jeep when I was in Germany. I'd have gone to Russia. Maybe that'd make the Pennsylvania papers.

N–2. Would you like that? [*Encouraging evaluation.*]

P–3. I wanted to be somebody in the Army. I could have been a Kamikaze pilot for the U.S. Army if I'd had enough education.

Fifth Hour

P–1. I don't want to see anything about coal mines on television. I know when I was drafted—June 27, 1941. I worked in the Ellbert mines with my oldest brother. What's all those visions in the kitchens for?

N–2. What kind of visions? [*Encouraging description of perceptions.*]

P–3. I don't know why they have me locked up in here. I wouldn't get lost in Pennsylvania. Why did I get lost in the United States after I got discharged?

N–4. Did you? Where? [*Exploring. The nurse gave a literal response here to an expression that had figurative meaning.*]

P–5. At home. I didn't like my people. The further away from home I got, the better I liked it.

Seventh Hour

P–1. I'll never get a privilege card. I have to live in the hospital for my skull. I want to sleep at night. I don't want to play with my penis. I don't want to weaken my heart and stomach and rectum.

N–2. Do you think it does that? [*Encouraging evaluation.*]

P–3. I don't know. If you count 10 fingers, will you go to sleep?

N–4. Why don't you sleep? [*Requesting an explanation. Not very helpful.*]

P–5. I like to sleep.

N–6. Does something keep you awake? [*Encouraging description of perceptions. More appropriate.*]

P–7. I don't know.

N–8. Sometimes worrying keeps people awake. [*Suggesting tentative meaning.*]

P–9. Worry? I wouldn't bother no civilians. I'd tell them about the brain surgical operation.

N–10. Do you worry at night? [*Exploring.*]

P–11. I don't know—I've had so many treatments, I don't know.

N–12. It's hard to think and remember things. [*Restating.*]

P–13. What makes you curse?

N–14. I guess getting angry. [*Suggesting tentative meaning.*]

P–15. Does a person get violent, disturbed, excited?

N–16. I guess he gets angry. [*Repeating.*]

P–17. Angry.

N–18. Do you feel this way sometimes? [*Encouraging evaluation.*]

P–19. Sometimes during the day.

N–20. Do you know what happens that results in your feeling angry? [*Encouraging description of perceptions.*]

P–21. No.

Eighth Hour

P–1. I want to be somebody in the United States.

N–2. Somebody important. [*Verbalizing the implied.*]

P–3. I want my name to be in the papers.

N–4. Why? [*Requesting an explanation. The nurse might ask, "What purpose would this serve?"*]

P–5. Since I was a kid, I wanted to do something for my parents.

P–6. Why weren't you in the bowling alley?

N–7. When? [*Seeking clarification.*]

P–8. Before the kill.

N–9. I didn't work here then. That was a long time ago. [*Giving information.*]

P–10. I'd like to go to a better ward. Do you think I have a penis in my mind?

N–11. How could that be? [*Encouraging description of perceptions.*]

P–12. I was thinking about that.

N–13. That'd be unusual, wouldn't it? [*Voicing doubt.*]

P–14. Yes, it would be unusual.

Eleventh Hour

P–1. As soon as I snap my fingers, I can see something on television. I wish I had a wife—a girl to write to. She's probably married to someone wasn't in the service at all. What do I have to live for?

N–2. Is it that you're concerned you won't be accepted when you leave the hospital? [*Suggesting tentative meaning.*]

P–3. Civilians are different people. There's some at home never was in the service.

N–4. How are civilians different? [*Encouraging comparison. Better worded "In what way. . . ?"*]

P–5. You got to stay out of your uniform many years to get acquainted with civilian people. That's rehabilitation.

Twelfth Hour

P–1. What do you get, 10 or 20 years for kill?

N–2. You're not sentenced; you're a patient. This isn't a prison; it's a hospital. [*Giving information.*]

(Pause. He put out his cigarette and ran his hands through his hair.)

N–3. You seem worried about something this morning. [*Verbalizing her observations.*]

P–4. I don't get any letters. Does alcoholism affect your heart? Make you mentally ill? Make you do things you shouldn't?

N–5. Sometimes. [*Giving information.*]

P–6. That's why I was drinking in Europe.

N–7. Why? [*Requesting an explanation. He has indicated that he knows why.*]

P–8. So I wouldn't worry.

N–9. What didn't you want to worry about? [*Exploring.*]

P–10. I didn't worry about the United States. I found a home in Germany.

P–11. I think I was born crazy.

N–12. Born crazy? [*Restating.*]

P–13. My dad scared his wife. Would that have something to do with pregnancy?

N–14. People used to think that. Now doctors feel that what makes a person sick is what happens to a person and how he feels about what happens to him. [*Giving information.*]

Study 6. *MR. F. E.* ______

An Hour with an Autistic Patient

The patient, aged 30, is the younger of two children. The father never supported the family. During the patient's early years, the father was in prison for robbery. Since the patient was four years old, his father has been hospitalized in a mental institution, following an attempt to murder his wife. From ages 4 to 11, the patient was in a very strict Polish orphanage. After that he lived with his mother near the San Francisco waterfront. At 16 he quit school in the tenth grade. In August, 1945, he was drafted, sent overseas to Germany, and hospitalized—all within six months. After a year in an Army hospital, he was admitted to a Veterans Administration hospital, where he has spent the last 10 years.

P–1. I'm as old as the world.[1]

N–2. You feel as old as the world? [*Attempting to translate into feelings.*]

P–3. I feel as old as the world. I go out in the waterfront and swim out there for 'em.

N–4. Whom do you have to swim for? [*Exploring. However, the nurse gave a literal response to a statement of figurative meaning.*]

P–5. Any of them children—drains out in the ocean. You understand?

N–6. Not exactly. [*Seeking clarification.*]

P–7. You're looking at a human being, you know, that's out of this world.

N–8. How can you be out of this world? [*Encouraging description of perceptions. Perhaps better worded, "In what way are you. . . ."*]

P–9. When you live out in the ocean, you're out of this world.

[1] The following verbal exchange is reprinted with permission from Hays, Joyce Samhammer: "Focusing on Feelings," *Nursing Outlook,* **10**:332–33, May 1962.

N–10. Is that where you want to be? [*Encouraging evaluation.*]

P–11. No, no. That's where I am. I live out there. I get outside there. How I get out there I'll never know. You can never know how you get your freedom. It's all finished and done. It's the same old ocean story—all people include all people.

N–12. What does that mean? [*Seeking clarification. Perhaps better worded, "I don't follow you."*]

P–13. They're all looking at me—I don't know how I'll come out of it.

N–14. Out of what? [*Seeking clarification.*]

P–15. When they all looks at me—that's as old as the world. It includes them all—that's the way they live in the world. I have to make my own way of living.

N–16. What way is that? [*Encouraging description.*]

P–17. That's a thing I'll never find out. I got my little grass place out there—I'm a loser in everything—there's always someone better than me.

N–18. Why are you a loser? [*Requesting an explanation. Perhaps the nurse could say, "You've never felt that there was anything you could do well."*]

P–19. I'll never be a winner. I live for everybody—because it's the best way of living. If I stay out of people's lives, I'll be better off—out in the ocean.

N–20. Why? [*Requesting an explanation. The nurse might have asked, "In what way will you be better off?" or "Will you really be happy that way?"*]

P–21. I likes to stay out of people's lives. I feel sorry for them—I'm useless.

N–22. You're not any good? [*Restating.*]

P–23. No, I'll never be any good in this world. All people know everything about everything—they play any kind of game they want. They play them games and are forgotten in the world.

N–24. Are *you* forgotten? [*Reflecting.*]

P–25. I'm forgotten and everything, but I like to see the wind blowing. I'm as old as Adam and Eve. I got no race, name, or nothing.

N–26. No name? [*Restating.*]

P–27. I ain't hot or cold—I ain't nothing. I'se just a useless neighborhood kid. I couldn't find nothing in this world. You got to keep out of trouble—the way I does it is keep them out of my life. The world is made to live and play in the world. The ocean is out of the world—nobody understands me.

N–28. Why can't they? [*Requesting an explanation. Not too helpful.*]

P–29. I just wouldn't know why.

N–30. What can't they understand about you? [*Exploring. This is more useful. Encouraging description.*]

P–31. I don't know—they can't understand—what kind of human being I am or anything.

N–32. What kind of human being are you? [*Encouraging evaluation and description.*]

P–33. I just can't understand what kind I am. I'm living, that's all. I'm satisfied—I *was* satisfied. It's to live and play in the world—that's the way they like it—to stay out of their lives. Me—I like them to have their freedom. I loves my own people—they're separated and unassociated. They want anything off me they can have it.

N–34. But aren't you all alone that way? [*Attempting to translate into feelings.*]

P–35. Yeah—yeah. (Spoken softly.)

N–36. Isn't it lonely? [*Attempting to translate into feelings.*]

P–37. Yeah, but I likes an empty room. The world's made to live and play in.

N–38. Is that what you're doing? [*Reflecting.*]

P–39. No.

N–40. Why can't you live in the world? [*Requesting an explanation. She could ask, "What seems to prevent you from. . . ?"*]

P–41. I don't know—it's separated and unassociated—I can't understand people—I just don't know how they live in this world.

N–42. Do they live different than you do? [*Encouraging comparison.*]

P–43. Yeah, that's the way they likes to live. I likes everybody to live in this world—I lives out of this world.

N–44. Couldn't you live in the world, too? [*Exploring.*]

P–45. I could, but I don't.

N–46. Why not? [*Requesting an explanation. Not helpful technique. If the patient knew these things, he probably wouldn't be sick.*]

P–47. I wouldn't know why.

N–48. You feel "different"? [*Suggesting tentative meaning.*]

P–49. Yeah.

N–50. You don't know how you're different. [*Accepting. Better worded, ". . . in what way you're different."*]

P–51. No, I just don't know how people could live that way and forget them. I don't want nothing off of nobody.

N–52. You mean you don't want to be a bother. [*Verbalizing the implied. Better worded, "You're saying that you don't want to be a bother."*]

P–53. That's the way I feel about it.

N–54. You want to take care of yourself. [*Restating. Accepting.*]

P–55. (He nodded.)

Even though the patient uses autistic language, his feelings are relatively clear to the nurse after just one hour. It is obvious that he feels isolated, lonely, rejected, useless, different, without identity, and a failure in living.

Study 7. TOMMY M. ______
Interaction on a Pediatric Unit

The patient, aged 11, had rheumatic fever.

N–1. How do you like being in the hospital? [*Encouraging evaluation. Better worded, "What are your feelings about being in the hospital?"*]

P–2. It's okay. Get out of doing schoolwork.

N–3. How did you feel when you were told you had to come to the hospital? [*Encouraging description. "What were your feelings when. . . ?"*]

P–4. I wanted to stay home.

N–5. Don't you like the hospital? [*Encouraging evaluation but assuming that negative feelings exist. Expressing what seems to be disapproval or surprise at such an idea.*]

P–6. Yeah. The nurses are okay too.

N–7. Do you know why you're in the hospital? [*Testing.*]

P–8. Yeah. I got rheumatic fever or something.

N–9. What are you making? [*Introducing a new topic. Expressing interest in what the patient is doing.*]

P–10. Puppets out of tissue. Wait till my mom finds out I used my whole box of tissues.

N–11. What gave you the idea? [*Exploring. The nurse had an opportunity to explore the mother-child relationship. She might have asked, "What do you think she'll say?"*]

P–12. I don't know. It's just something to do.

P–13. What's that?

N–14. It's just something I'm writing about you. [*Giving information. This is vague. The nurse could say, "I'm writing down what you and I say."*]

N–15. Does it bother you to have someone write something about you? [*Encouraging evaluation but suggesting negative feelings.*]

P–16. Yeah, I thought it was like a psychiatrist or something.

N–17. Why? Didn't you ever have anyone write something about you? [*Requesting an explanation. Encouraging comparison of the nurse's behavior with that of others.*]

N–18. Do you know which part of your body is sick? [*Testing to see what he knows about his illness. The nurse gives no information when the patient indicates that he lacks this knowledge.*]

P–19. No, my mother didn't tell me.

N–20. Do you mind staying in bed? [*Encouraging evaluation but again suggesting negative feelings.*]

P–21. Not really. Get bored.

N–22. You don't mind someone else washing you and doing everything for you? [*Requesting his evaluation but indicating that he should feel uncomfortable being dependent on others.*]
(No response.)

N–23. How do you like the food? [*Introducing another topic for him to evaluate.*]

P–24. It's okay.

N–25. How much longer are you going to stay in the hospital? [*Testing. The wording implies that the decision is his to make.*]

P–26. Another week.

N–27. Did the doctor tell you that? [*Exploring.*]

P–28. No, but I figured it out.

N–29. What are you going to do this summer? [*Introducing another new and unrelated topic.*]

P–30. Go to Atlantic City.

N–31. I'll bet that's fun. [*Expressing her own opinion.*]

It is interesting to note that the nurse does not call the patient by name, nor does she tell him her name. All topics were initiated by the nurse, who primarily asked direct questions. At no time was the patient encouraged to take the initiative and discuss what might have been of concern or of interest to him. At the end, the nurse seems to leave without comment or explanation—just as she had entered.

Study 8. JOHNNY S.

Interaction on a Pediatric Unit

The patient, aged 8, had infectious mononucleosis.

N–1. You don't like staying in bed, do you? [*Encouraging a negative evaluation. An abrupt beginning.*]

P–2. You've got the answer.

N–3. Why don't you like staying in bed? [*Requesting an explanation.*]

P–4. Don't know, but it sure is awful.

N–5. Awful, why? [*Restating. Requesting an explanation. Better worded, "In what way. . . ?"*]

P–6. Only thing I can do is make a mess. Get everything wet. There's a leak in the rag.

(The patient was playing with water in a cup—trying to put water into a paper with a tongue blade.)

N–7. You're really having a hard time. [*Reflecting. It is noteworthy that the nurse was accepting and expressed no disapproval.*]

P–8. You're not kidding.

(His television set was playing.)

N–9. What's on TV? [*Introducing a new topic. Expressing interest in what he may be watching.*]

P–10. Burns and Allen.

N–11. Do you like that? [*Encouraging evaluation.*]

(No answer.)

P–12. I know one thing. I'm getting all dirty.

N–13. What happens when your nurse finds this? [*Encouraging description of what he expects.*]

P–14. No nurse is taking care of me today.

N–15. You like a nurse to take care of you. [*Verbalizing what the nurse feels is implied.*]

P–16. Yeah!

N–17. What does the nurse do when she takes care of you? [*Encouraging description.*]

P–18. I don't know.

(The patient in the next bed made a puppet for him and gave it to him.)

N–19. What's the puppet's name? [*Exploring.*]

P–20. I don't know.

(He cleaned up all the water from the table and floor with tissues.)

P–21. I hope I'll be going home soon—in six or eight weeks.

N–22. Why six or eight weeks? [*Requesting an explanation.*]

P–23. 'Cause that's what the doctor said.

N–24. How about school? [*Introducing a new topic.*]

P–25. No more school. It's summer.

N–26. What about the school you missed? [*Exploring.*]

P–27. I know something gooder than my boy friend. I passed third grade without taking exams.

(He suddenly noticed the writing the nurse was doing.)

P–28. Hey, what's that you're writing?

N–29. A story. [*Giving misinformation.*]

P–30. What's the name?

N–31. Oh, I don't know. What do you think it should be? [*Evading. Reflecting question back to him.*]

P–32. It's your story.

N–33. Think you'll have to stay in bed all the time in the hospital? [*Testing.*]

P–34. Yep, I know it.

N–35. How do you feel about it? [*Encouraging evaluation. "What are your feelings. . . ?"*]

P–36. Awful!

N–37. Awful? [*Restating.*]

P–38. 'Course. Have to stay in bed. I'm allowed out of bed in the room but not in the hall. [*It would seem that he is more concerned about the relative isolation than the inactivity.*]

P–39. May I have a piece of paper to draw?

N–40. Sure. What will you draw? [*Complying. Exploring. Encouraging description.*]

P–41. A good person—an old person—a funny person. My mother taught me how to draw it.

(He drew a human figure, which was far out of proportion.)

P–42. It's a clown.

N–43. Do you like clowns? [*Encouraging evaluation. A more revealing question might have been, "What are clowns like? What kind of people are they?"*]

P–44. Yeah.

N–45. Where did you see clowns? [*Exploring.*]

P–46. In a circus.

N–47. They're fun, aren't they? [*Expressing an opinion. Anticipating his agreement.*]

P–48. Had a circus in the school yard. Had clowns and a ferris wheel.

N–49. Did you ever see a circus with wild animals? [*Exploring related aspect of the topic.*]

P–50. Yeah, my father took me. Look what my girl friend sent me.

(He showed the nurse a get-well card with five dimes attached.)

N–51. That's very nice. [*Giving approval.*]

P–52. Last time I was here she sent me 10 dimes.

N–53. She must be rich. [*Expressing an exaggerated opinion.*]

P–54. She is. I'm writing a story.

N–55. What does it say? [*Encouraging description.*]

P–56. I don't know; I'm just writing it.

(He was copying the words from the front of a comic book.)

N–57. When were you in the hospital? [*Placing event in time.*]

P–58. About five months.

N–59. You mean five months ago? [*Seeking consensual validation. Better worded, "Are you saying five. . . ?"*]

P–60. From the last time I left to now is five months.

N–61. Why were you here last time? [*Requesting an explanation. The nurse might ask, "What was your problem?"*]

P–62. Because of stomach aches. That's why I'm here now.

N–63. You got better so you went home? [*Verbalizing the implied. The nurse covered a lot of ground that might have been more fully explored; e.g., she might say, "Tell me what this was like and what your feelings were about all this."*]

P–64. Yep.

N–65. I bet you were happy to go home. [*Verbalizing the implied.*]

P–66. Uh hmm!

N–67. What happened when Mommy said you had to come back? [*Encouraging description.*]

P–68. Got me mad!

N–69. Got you mad? [*Restating.*]
(No answer.)

N–70. Why mad? [*Requesting an explanation. She might say, "Tell me about this feeling."*]
(Still no response.)

P–71. I'm busy writing my story.

N–72. Okay, I'll leave you now. [*Accepting. Giving information.*]

P–73. 'Bye.

9. *MR. JOSEPH W.* — *A Neurologic Patient*

The patient had hemiplegia following brain injury.

Friday

N–1. Hello, Joe, how are you feeling today? [*Encouraging evaluation. Better worded, "What are your feelings?" or "What would you say your mood is today?"*]

P–2. I feel with my hands like I always do.

N–3. You know what I mean, Joe. Seriously, how are you today? [*Encouraging evaluation.*]

P–4. Okay, I guess. As well as can be expected. What do you care?

N–5. Okay, Joe, I'll go if you want me to. See you later. [*Expressing disapproval by withdrawing. She might say, "You feel my interest is not sincere?"*]

P–6. I didn't ask you to go. But I get sick and tired of students coming up to me and saying (mimicking), "Hello, how do you feel?"

N–7. I know what you mean—guess it does get sort of monotonous. [*Accepting.*]

P–8. Why do you have that bandage on your ankle?

N–9. I burnt it. [*Giving information.*]

P–10. How?

N–11. On the cylinder of a motorcycle. I didn't get off right, but I know better now. [*Giving information.*]

P–12. I have a 'cycle at home. I wonder if it's still there.

N–13. What kind do you have? [*Exploring.*]

P–14. Harley Davis.

N–15. So do I—that is, it's Bill's, the fellow I'm engaged to. He keeps it as a hobby and can take it apart and put it together blindfolded. [*Giving information of a personal nature that the patient does not need.*]

P–16. I used to be able to do that. My wife really liked to ride with me. Have you ever gone to 'cycle races or shows?

N–17. No, I haven't; what are they like? [*Encouraging description.*]

P–18. Nice. I was the clown at the shows and did crazy stunts. I did headstands on the seat of the 'cycle while doing about 95 to 100 miles an hour.

N–19. Wow! I'll bet you stole the show. [*Expressing surprise. Giving approval.*]

P–20. Yeah.

N–21. Say, Bill has a lot of magazines on 'cycles, races, and national events. Would you like some, Joe? [*Offering something concrete.*]

P–22. No, you'll only forget them and I'll be disappointed.

N–23. No, you won't. I'll bring them Monday. [*Giving information.*]

Monday

(The nurse approached the patient with the magazines. He leaned out of his bed with his hand extended.)

N–1. Here they are, Joe. [*Giving something concrete.*]

P–2. I thought you'd forget.

(Nurse and patient thumbed through some of the magazines, commenting and pointing out pictures to each other.)

P–3. Will you do me a favor this afternoon, if you've time, nurse?

N–4. Sure, what is it? [*Offering self.*]

P–5. Write a letter to my wife for me?

N–6. I'd be glad to, Joe. I'll be back after class. [*Offering concrete assistance. Giving information.*]

P–7. You won't forget, will you?

N–8. No, I won't forget. [*Reassuring.*]

(The nurse found out later that the letter she wrote for him that afternoon was one of many the patient sent to his wife. None is ever answered.)

Tuesday

P–1. Do you love this guy you're going to marry?

N–2. Of course, I do, Joe. [*Giving information.*]

P–3. Does he love you?

N–4. Yes. [*Giving information. When the patient uses the time to interview the nurse about personal matters, the nurse can state that she cannot see the value to him of such discussion and suggest that they use the time to explore his problems.*]

P–5. You'll never know if he does—'cause you can't read anyone's mind, and some day after you're married, he'll walk out on you. What would you think? What would you do if it did happen?

N–6. I don't think it will. [*Offering an opinion that keeps the conversation focused on her. It would appear that the patient is expressing feelings about his own marriage. The nurse might ask, "Is this the way it was for you?"*]

P–7. A part of you dies, that's what happens.

N–8. I know what you mean, Joe. I guess it does. [*Accepting. She might add, "Would you care to tell me about it?"*]

P–9. Well, you take my advice and build your coffin now, because it will happen.

N–10. It takes all kinds of people to make up a world and everybody's different. [*Making a stereotyped comment. Her intention is to imply that not all relationships are disappointing, not all persons are untrustworthy. She might say, "You seem to feel that marriage inevitably results in unhappiness."*]

(The patient changed the subject back to motor cycles. Later.)

N–11. It's time for me to leave. I'll see you in the morning.

P–12. Okay. Don't oversleep and be late for work.

Although much of the conversation was of a social nature, this relationship, as it progressed, did achieve much of its aim. As the student nurse expressed it, "As the result of an accident, Mr. W., a long-term neurologic patient, has been severed from all the normal contacts and functions of everyday life because of his hemiplegia. Having been hurt many times in the past, he has built up a shell around himself—outwardly displaying a picture of bitterness, cynicism, and sarcasm. He makes some effort to hide this by gibing everyone from this vantage point—distrusting, suspicious, the world his 'enemy.' When he was shown some interest, he was afraid of being disappointed, as he had apparently been many times before. Therefore, he met this offer with morose and sarcastic replies. At the same time, he snatches at any kindness or attention in an almost selfish way and gives nothing in return. The only way I can see to help this patient at this time is to be consistent with warmth, interest, and understanding."

Study 10. MRS. A. F. ______

Relating to the Patient in Labor

The patient was a primipara.

N–1. How are you doing? [*Encouraging evaluation. This is vague, as is the patient's answer. The nurse seems to be asking the patient to evaluate her own progress, while the patient may well expect such a judgment to come from the professional staff. The nurse might ask, "Are you comfortable?"*]

P–2. Okay, I guess.

N–3. How far apart are your pains? [*Seeking information.*]

P–4. About every seven or eight minutes.

N–5. Tell me when your next one begins; I'll time it. [*Encouraging description of perceptions. Giving information.*]

P–6. All right.

N–7. What's it going to be—a boy or a girl? [*Asking an unrealistic question.*]

P–8. A boy.

P–9. The pain is starting.

N–10. That one lasted 45 seconds. [*Giving information, based on her observations.*]

P–11. They're getting pretty bad.

N–12. You're doing fine. What name have you picked for the baby? [*Reassuring. Introducing an unrelated topic.*]

P–13. Jonathan.

N–14. That's nice—I like that. [*Giving approval.*]

P–15. My husband selected it.

N–16. What if it's a girl? [*Exploring.*]

P–17. It won't be—we want a boy too badly.

N–18. I'm going to take your blood pressure. [*Introducing an unrelated topic. Giving information.*]

P–19. Is it all right?

N–20. It's fine. [*Reassuring.*]

P–21. Tell me, are many babies born abnormal—deformed?

N–22. No, why do you ask? [*Giving information. Requesting an explanation.*]

P–23. I just wondered.

N–24. I have to go now. Is there anything I can get for you? [*Giving information. Offering assistance of a vague nature, after implying that she has little or no time left to devote to the patient.*]

P–25. I guess not. Will I be alone in here?

N–26. I'll be nearby if you want anything. [*Giving information that is intended to be reassuring.*]

The patient is obviously quite anxious. The nurse, finding no evidence that the patient is in need of further physical care, withdraws without exploring the patient's psychologic needs, many of which were suggested by the content of the patient's questions and responses.

Study 11. MRS. P.

Excerpts from a Delivery Room Discussion Immediately Postpartum

P–1. Can I have this blood pressure thing off my arm?

N–2. You had better wait awhile. [*Giving advice. Perhaps the nurse could say, "Not just yet."*]

(The patient moans.)

N–3. You seem to be moaning, Mrs. P. [*Making an observation.*]

P–4. Why do they have me on this hard table all alone?

N–5. Are you uncomfortable? [*Evading patient's question. Encouraging evaluation.*]

(No response.) [*It would seem, however, that the patient is quite obviously uncomfortable. The nurse might say, "I'll be here with you. It must be uncomfortable for you." She could then give information that would indicate the reason for the patient's being there.*]

N–6. You look like you're deep in thought. [*Making an observation.*]

P–7. No, just sleepy. The doctor took blood from my arm.

N–8. Were you frightened? [*Encouraging evaluation but suggesting negative feelings.*]

P–9. No, I was relaxed, but it hurt. How many days do they keep you in here?

N–10. About four or five. [*Giving information.*]

P–11. That's what I thought. (Sighs.)

N–12. Do you mind staying? [*Encouraging evaluation but again suggesting a negative response. Better worded, "What are your feelings about staying?"*]

P–13. I'm worried about my children.

N–14. Is anyone with them? [*Exploring.*]

P–15. My oldest daughter. Look how slow this bottle is dripping. I guess it will be midnight before it's done. I would like it to be over.

P–16. Everybody will be surprised. I wasn't supposed to have this baby until August.

N–17. I guess it was a surprise to you, too. [*Tentatively suggesting what may have been the patient's feelings.*]

P–18. I could tell—when you've had enough kids, you can usually tell. I don't know how much she weighed; I only heard her crying. They just leave you in here and forget you until they happen to walk by. [*Patient is indicating that she has unmet needs about which the personnel seem unconcerned. Perhaps she feels that no one cares about her as a person. In addition, she is concerned about the condition of her baby, which was more than a month premature.*]

(The patient rubs her abdomen.)

N–19. I see you are rubbing your stomach. [*Making an observation.*]

P–20. It feels so good to be flat.

(A nurse came in to tell Mrs. P. that the baby weighed five pounds, eight ounces.)

N–21. Do you feel better now? [*Encouraging evaluation but seeming to imply that this information is sufficient to meet all the patient's needs.*]

P–22. Yes.

(The patient went to sleep.)

12. *MRS. L.*

Interaction with a New Mother

The patient had had a caesarean section. This was the third postoperative day.

N–1. You seem to be having some pain. [*Making an observation.*]

P–2. No pain. It's just the tape pulling.

N–3. Have you been walking around yet? [*Introducing a topic for conversation.*]

P–4. Oh, yes, I was up on my first day, walking from bed to chair. Nobody around here helps you.

N–5. Do you mean no one helps you to walk around? [*Seeking consensual validation. Perhaps if the nurse had asked, "No one helps you?" the patient might have verbalized her feelings more freely. "Do you mean" often has an intimidating effect.*]

P–6. Yes.
(Silence.)

N–7. Is this your first baby? [*Introducing a new topic.*]

P–8. No. My second living. I had two miscarriages. This is a boy.

N–9. He must be a cute little boy. [*Making a stereotyped comment. This is especially meaningless when she has not even seen the baby.*]

P–10. Oh, he's all right.
(Silence.)

P–11. I just want to tell you one thing—don't have a Caesarean. All it is is suffering.

N–12. I can understand that you would have some pain. We've already had our maternity experience, and we were with many mothers in your position. [*Belittling the patient's feelings by implying that she is in no way* *unique. The nurse might say, "It was a painful experience; perhaps you'd like to tell me about it."*]

P–13. Oh, yes? Well, I feel better now. I'll be glad when Monday comes and I have my stitches out. It's a lot to go through, having a baby. No more for me.

N–14. You must have had a hard time with the baby. [*The nurse noted, "I felt she was blaming the baby for the discomfort she experienced." Verbalizing the implied. Seeming to indicate acceptance, yet feeling disapproval.*]

P–15. Well, I was afraid when they told me I had to have a Caesarean. They put me to sleep, but I saw the baby come out of my stomach. Then they put that awful oxygen over my face. Before I had pain when my first baby was born. This time I had pain after the baby was born.

P–16. What are you doing anyway? I don't want to see what I'm telling you in the paper.

N–17. No, Mrs. L., you won't. We are students from ____ and we are in psychiatric nursing here at ____. We are just speaking to patients in other areas this afternoon. [*Giving information that obviously creates anxiety.*]

P–18. Oh, you think I'm sick in the head.

N–19. No, Mrs. L., we are talking to other patients—both to talk to them and to understand for ourselves how well we can talk with them. My notes are just for my own use. Your name is not on them, and I promise you, you'll never see them in the newspapers. [*Giving information that is somewhat vague in describing the purpose of nurses' interacting verbally with patients.*]

P–20. Oh, I see. Well, it's nice talking to you.

N–21. Well, Mrs. L., it's been pleasant sitting with you. I wish you good luck with the baby. I think you'll be a good mother. [*Expressing appreciation. Giving approval.*]

It would appear that both nurse and patient close with stereotyped comments, the sincerity of which is questionable.

Study 13. *MRS. J.* ______

Excerpts from a Discussion with a Surgical Patient

The patient was 50 years old.

[The nurse introduced herself, said she would like to talk with the patient, and asked how she felt.]

P–1. I just had an operation and I don't feel well. I wish it hadn't happened to me.

(The patient went on in detail explaining the operation.)

N–2. You talk about your operation a lot. I wonder how you feel. [*Making an observation. Encouraging evaluation. Better worded, "I wonder what your feelings are."*]

P–3. I feel sad. I came in here sick and I expected to be better now.

N–4. It must be hard to talk about this. [*Verbalizing the implied. Accepting.*]

P–5. It is. All these things started happening at once and I haven't been any good since.

N–6. I don't understand. [*Seeking clarification. Better worded, "I don't follow."*]

P–7. Well, it was one thing, then another. First, a lump in my breast, then they removed my ovary, and now this. I lived a good life and enjoyed myself. Everyone feels sad for me.

N–8. You say everyone is sad for you; are you sad too? [*Reflecting.*]

P–9. You can't enjoy activities or life when you're not normal. Nobody knows when they'll get struck down, but you have to expect it when you get old.

P–10. (Looking at her gastric and intravenous tubing.) I want to turn over, but I can't with all these tubes.

N–11. I don't think I'd like to lie in one position a long time. [*The nurse attempts to express her empathy, but in so doing may seem to be saying, "I'm glad that I'm not in your predicament." She focuses on her own feelings rather than on the patient's. Perhaps she could say, "You must be very uncomfortable." She might also alter the patient's position to the extent that this is possible without interfering with the tubing.*]

P–12. I'm not used to it. I always slept on my stomach, but now I can't. (Pause.) [The student nurse noted that she felt uncomfortable during the silence.]

(The patient appeared to be watching television. A visitor entered.)

N–13. I must leave now. Thank you, Mrs. J. [*Giving information. Expressing appreciation. It would seem that both nurse and patient welcomed the opportunity to terminate the conversation.*]

P–14. You're welcome.

As a first step, the nurse might help the patient to explore realistically the extent to which she will be handicapped by the surgery and the activities she still will be able to enjoy. Her feelings of not being "any good" and being "not normal" should also be discussed more fully.

14. *MR. R.*

Interaction with a Medical Patient

The patient, aged 66, was on the medical service.

N–1. Good morning, Mr. R. How are you today? [*Offering recognition. Encouraging evaluation.*]

P–2. I don't feel very well.

N–3. In what way? [*Encouraging description.*]

P–4. I just don't—I have trouble with my bowels.

N–5. You're constipated? [*Seeking consensual validation.*]

P–6. Yeah.

N–7. Do you sleep pretty well? [*Exploring other aspects of his health.*]

P–8. No, I don't. They give me sleeping pills.

N–9. Do the pills help? [*Encouraging evaluation.*]

P–10. They help some.

N–11. You feel pretty sad? [*Tentatively suggesting what she feels may be the patient's mood. Rather than suggest a particular feeling, the nurse might ask directly, "What would you say your mood is?"*]

P–12. I don't feel good, I just don't feel good at all.

N–13. What do you think the problem is? [*Reflecting—to encourage description from the patient's viewpoint.*]

P–14. This here constipation seems to be the worse.

N–15. If your bowels were better, do you think you'd feel better? [*Encouraging evaluation, trying to discover whether the patient sees this as his only problem. Again, she could ask this directly.*]

P–16. I don't know.

N–17. You've had this trouble for some time now? [*Exploring. Verbalizing what seems to be implied.*]

P–18. Yeah.

N–19. When did it all start? [*Attempting to place event in time.*]

P–20. Oh, I don't know really.

N–21. Very long ago? [*Attempting to place in time.*]

P–22. It was quite some time ago. They have it all on the chart. (The patient expelled gas orally several times.)

N–23. Does your stomach bother you too? [*Introducing a topic suggested by the patient's behavior.*]

P–24. Yes, it does. My whole insides. I've had several operations.

P–25. I've been trying to do the best I can—I'm way underweight.

N–26. You don't have much of an appetite, I guess. [*Suggesting a possible explanation—seeking confirmation.*]

P–27. Not too much. I do the best I can. [*The nurse might explore what it is he does.*]

N–28. Do you get any medicine during the day? [*Exploring.*]

P–29. Yes, they give me medicine.

N–30. Does it make you feel any different? [*Encouraging evaluation. Not too helpful unless the nurse knows what the medication is and its purpose.*]

P–31. I don't know that, nurse.

N–32. No difference that you can see. [*Verbalizing the implied.*]

P–33. No.

N–34. What do you think is the cause of all your trouble? [*Asking the patient if he can explain the source of his difficulties. It is unrealistic, at this time, to expect him to do so.*]

P–35. Well, I don't know, nurse.

N–36. Do you worry a lot? [*Introducing what—to the patient—is an unrelated topic.*]

P–37. I just feel bad.

N–38. Do you have any pain? [*Exploring.*]

P–39. It's just sort of misery—to feel bound up inside.

P–40. I really am sick, nurse. They feel it's my imagination.

N–41. Being sick is not imaginary. Worry can make your body sick. [*Giving information.*]

P–42. It's not worry that done it.

N–43. You don't feel that you worry a lot? [*The nurse seems to be disapproving of the patient's inability to accept anxiety as a source of his physical problems.*]

P–44. To make it short, I just feel bad.

N–45. What do you think might help? [*Reflecting. However, the patient may take this to mean that the professional personnel have no plans for his treatment.*]

P–46. I don't know whether I can answer that.

N–47. Do you have any ideas? [*Restating her previous question.*]

P–48. No, I don't.

N–49. We do want to help you. [*Offering information that is intended to be reassuring. What the patient is interested in is how and when he will receive help; he is not even sure that anyone understands the problem.*]

P–50. I know. I realize that.

P–51. I'd like to rest awhile now.

N–52. All right. [*Accepting.*]

The nurse has attempted to cause the patient to become aware of a relationship between his emotional problems and his physical symptoms in the course of a single conversation. When she is unsuccessful, she seems unsure as to how to proceed.

Study 15. *MR. K.* ______

Excerpts from a Discussion with a Patient Admitted for Medical Observation

N–1. Hello, Mr. K. I'm Miss C. I'm a nurse at____. May I speak to you for a bit? [*Giving information. Offering recognition.*]

P–2. Sure, sure. Sit down.

N–3. Thank you. How are you feeling? [*Encouraging evaluation. Perhaps better worded, "What are your feelings about being in the hospital?" Or if it is the patient's physical condition she is concerned about, she might ask whether he is comfortable.*]

P–4. Very well, thank you. I'm not too sick, as you can see.

N–5. I'm glad to hear that you feel well. [*Giving approval. The nurse might say, "You appear to be comfortable at the present."*]

P–6. Yes, I'm here for observation—low blood pressure—isn't painful or anything—it's just like being at home. I keep busy. I'm a ____ inspector and can do my work here, so I never get bored.

N–7. Do you think a hospital would be boring if you didn't have these things to occupy your time? [*Reflecting. Exploring the "boredom" that he seemed to imply might occur in a hospital.*]

P–8. Yes, boring and depressing, of course. Sick people all around. There aren't many well people in a hospital, (laughing) except the nurses, of course.

N–9. What about the nurses, how do you feel about them? [*Encouraging evaluation and description of perceptions. Better worded, "What are your feelings. . . ?"*]

P–10. I think they must be hard-hearted.

N–11. Hard-hearted? I don't understand what you mean. Could you explain? [*Restating. Seeking clarification. Better worded, "I don't follow what you're saying. Could you tell me more about this?"*]

P–12. Well, I think it's just like a piece of meat or something. You know, forget about the person, just concentrate on the injury.

N–13. Have you come across any nurses who do this? [*Exploring. It is worth noting that the nurse feels secure enough to avoid defending the nursing profession.*]

P–14. Yes, quite a few.

N–15. How does it make you feel? [*Encouraging evaluation. Better worded, "What are your feelings about this?"*]

P–16. I'm not sure. Sometimes I get pretty mad. I don't like feeling unimportant.

N–17. I don't blame you. I think I might feel the same. Tell me, have you any other feelings about nurses? [*Accepting. Indicating absence of disapproval. Exploring.*]

P–18. I've always wondered if some nurses don't enjoy giving I.M.'s (A practical nurse took the patient's temperature, pulse, and respirations and left.)

P–19. See what I mean; they're hard-hearted. Not even a smile. I bet she'll smile about 11 o'clock tonight.

N–20. Why do you think that? [*Requesting an explanation. Better worded, "What has happened to give you that impression?"*]

P–21. She'll be glad to leave.

N–22. I can understand how you might feel that she doesn't enjoy her work, especially if she appears so solemn. [*Accepting.*]

N–23. Well, I'm afraid our hour is up. Thank you for your time. Through things you've said I'll be better able to know how patients will respond to the hospital situation—that way, I'll be able not only to care for them physically, but I'll be able to understand their feelings, too. [*Giving information. Expressing appreciation.*]

P–24. I'm glad you came. 'Bye and thanks.

Study 16. MR. FRED G.

A Relationship with a Patient on an Admission Service

The patient, 29 years of age, is the oldest of four siblings. The patient is described as having a close relationship with his mother and a negative one with his father. He was considered erratic in his studies and completed only the first year of high school. A teacher described him as "extremely nervous, but of calm appearance." He enlisted in the Army when he was 19 and saw active duty in Korea as a medical aidman. He was honorably discharged in 1953 and made a poor social adjustment as a civilian. On his first admission to the hospital in February, 1961, the physician described his complaints as "inability to concentrate, feelings of depersonalization, alienation from his environment, and obsessive rumination." Just prior to the beginning of this relationship, the patient was described as "preoccupied, tense, anxious, pacing up and down the hall."

Mr. G. is a patient on the admission service. As the nurse entered the dayroom, she observed, "The patient was stretched out on two chairs, disheveled-looking, eyes closed. The nursing supervisor and I walked over and stood by his chair until he opened his eyes to look at us. After the supervisor introduced me to the patient and left, I said 'Hello' and asked whether I could talk with him. He nodded 'yes.' He agreed that I could write down our conversation, having been reassured that he could see what I wrote at any time."

First Hour

N–1. I'd like to talk with you several times a week; I'd like to help you help yourself. [*Giving information about the relationship. Offering self.*]

P–2. It's a good idea.

N–3. How do you feel today? [*Encouraging evaluation. Better worded, "What are your feelings today?"*]

P–4. Good mood.

N–5. Could you explain what you mean so that I could understand what you mean? [*Seeking clarification. Seeking consensual validation of "good mood." "Explain" and "mean" are intimidating words. The nurse might say, "Tell me what you're saying in greater detail so that I can grasp this."*]

P–6. I'm resting easy, comfortable, and feeling cheerful.

N–7. I don't think you look cheerful. [*Making an observation. A less-negative observation might be, "To me you appear less than cheerful."*]

P–8. I am more cheerful than I've been. What else do you want to know?

N–9. What do you want to tell me? [*Reflecting. Giving a broad opening.*]

P–10. I'm getting fine treatment. The nursing assistants and nurses are very nice—doctors give me a lot of attention.

N–11. You look sleepy. [*Making an observation.*]

P–12. Well, I have a backache.

N–13. Tell me about it. [*Exploring. Encouraging description.*]

P–14. It saps my strength, makes me uncomfortable.

N–15. In what way? [*Seeking clarification.*]

(The patient excused himself to go to the latrine. He returned shortly.)

P–16. I have this backache—it's a sprain—makes me uncomfortable.

N–17. In what way? [*Repeating her previous question. Seeking clarification.*]

P–18. Well, I have to do a lot of walking. I can't get comfortable in chairs.

N–19. Is it constant? [*Exploring.*]

P–20. Yes, constant pain.

N–21. Does it keep you awake? [*Exploring.*]

P–22. Yes.

N–23. When did you first get this? [*Attempting to place event in time.*]

P–24. Three years ago.

N–25. What were you doing when you first noticed this? [*Encouraging description.*]

P–26. Laboring work.

N–27. What kind? [*Exploring.*]

P–28. Lifting brick.

N–29. Are you a bricklayer by trade? [*Seeking clarification.*]

P–30. Yes.

N–31. Did you try other kinds of work? [*Exploring.*]

P–32. Counterman's work in a luncheonette.

N–33. Did your back ache then? [*Encouraging comparison.*]

P–34. Yes.

N–35. Have you had treatment? [*Exploring.*]

P–36. No. Oh, yes—x-ray—they didn't do anything.

N–37. How do you feel emotionally about this? [*Encouraging expression of feelings. Better worded, "What are your feelings. . . ?"*]

P–38. It upsets me emotionally.

N–39. Do you feel this is your entire problem? [*Reflecting. Encouraging evaluation. A timely question.*]

P–40. No.

N–41. Would you like to tell me more? I'd like to help you—why don't you just keep talking. [*Giving a broad opening. Offering self.*]

P–42. I don't know what to say.

N–43. You say this backache is not your entire problem. [*Restating.*]

P–44. No. I suffer from the memory of my combat days. I want to commit suicide—and also I hear voices.

N–45. What do they say? [*Encouraging description, but the nurse let her curiosity show and completely overlooked the most important revelation, "I want to commit suicide." Worth exploring later.*]

P–46. All sorts of things. I am very uncomfortable with my back—I keep wanting to kill myself.

N–47. Why—do you understand why you feel this way? [*Requesting an explanation. The nurse could ask, "What prompted this idea?"*]

P–48. Memory of combat days—I can't watch combat pictures or I crack up and cry.

N–49. Where did you have combat? [*Exploring.*]

P–50. Korea.

N–51. Would you like to talk about it? [*Giving a broad opening. Less likely to receive negative response if worded, "Tell me about your experience."*]

P–52. I was a medical aidman—handled about 20 wounded and about 10 men died in my time—and handling them took something out of me—

I wasn't the same type of man after that. [*What did it take out of him? In what way was he different?*]

N–53. Did this happen over a long period of time or at one clip? [*Exploring.*]

P–54. One clip—I was shocked to a degree.

N–55. This would be difficult for anyone. Anyone else there to help you? [*Accepting feelings expressed. Exploring.*]

P–56. Yes—a litter bearer.

N–57. How did it happen—an explosion? [*Encouraging description. The nurse should have asked, however, "What happened?" rather than "how," and the answer shouldn't have been suggested—this is just hitting in the dark.*]

P–58. Going out on patrol. It happened gradually—one clip—about 30-day period. I am being treated fine here. The hospital is good.

N–59. When a medical aide, what was your assignment? [*Getting him back on the subject. Exploring.*]

P–60. Go on patrol with men—group combat—and where there was action, I took care of the wounded.

N–61. Some of the experiences were rather rough. [*Accepting. Acknowledging that it was a difficult situation.*]

P–62. Yes.

N–63. I'd like to hear about the actual cases if you could tell me. [*Exploring.*]

P–64. Well (pause) don't remember too much. [*Somewhat contradictory, since it's the memories that he says bothers him.*]

N–65. You felt pretty bad when these men died? [*Encouraging evaluation.*]

P–66. Yeah, I'm very nervous—everyone was nervous.

N–67. Were you injured? [*Exploring.*]

P–68. I suffered combat fatigue.

N–69. Were you hospitalized? [*Exploring.*]

P–70. No.

N–71. Were you treated in any way? [*Exploring.*]

P–72. No, I am being treated here. Got the backache later in civilian life. [*There is more to the suicidal intent then than ridding himself of the back pain.*]

N–73. Who diagnosed the combat fatigue? [*Exploring.*]

P–74. I did.

N–75. When were you in Korea? [*Exploring. Attempting to place event in time.*]

P–76. 1953.

N–77. Were you relieved from duty? [*Exploring.*]

P–78. No—discharged.

N–79. You did very good work. [*Verbalizing the implied. This might be misinterpreted as approval. Better worded, "Am I correct in assuming that you feel your work was good?"*]

P–80. Yes, I did.

N–81. But now you think about it a great deal. [*Restating previously made comment to encourage further expression.*]

P–82. Yes. (Excused himself to get a cigarette light.) Since then, I've tried to commit suicide half a dozen times—tried gas, hanging, etc.

N–83. Because the memories haunt you? [*Restating for confirmation.*]

P–84. (Nodded "yes.")

N–85. When you say "memories," what flashes through your mind? [*Encouraging description. Most appropriate.*]

P–86. The dead men—men that died.

N–87. You were there to help, and you did all you could. [*Reassuring. The nurse does not really know, and he knows that she was not there. She might have said, "The men were beyond help?"*]

P–88. I know, but that's the way it affected me.

N–89. Did others who were with you feel this way? [*Exploring. Perhaps this is unrealistic. It is unlikely that he could know.*]

P–90. I don't know, but I know they suffered combat fatigue.

N–91. Would you like to feel different about this? [*Encouraging evaluation. This wording encourages a conventional reply. The nurse might ask, "The feeling you have is not one you want to have, is that it?"*]

P–92. Yes.

N–93. Do you have any idea how you can change this feeling? [*Encouraging the formulation of a plan of action. Somewhat early for this.*]

P–94. Well, they are teaching me here at the hospital to forget it. [*Is this what he wants to do?*]

N–95. How? [*Seeking clarification.*]

P–96. I don't know—occupy myself with different thoughts.

(The nurse got up to get a chair to prop the patient's feet on.)

P–97. Don't go away, come right back.

N–98. Does talking about this make you feel better? [*Encouraging evaluation.*]

P–99. Yeah.

N–100. Others have had these experiences. [*Belittling the feelings expressed.*] [*Perhaps this would have been a good time to stop, summarize, and then talk more about the purpose of the relationship.*]

(No response. The patient appeared to be getting restless.)

N–101. You're a chain smoker. [*Making an observation.*]

(The patient smiled a bit.) [The nurse noted that the smile was quite a change from the depressed expression.]

N–102. Do you have a family? [*Introducing a topic.*]

P–103. Mother, Father, two sisters, and brother.

N–104. Do they live nearby? [*Exploring.*]

P–105. New York.

N–106. Do they come to see you? [*Exploring.*]

P–107. Yes.

N–108. Would you like me to come again? [*Encouraging evaluation.*]

P–109. Yes. It's done me a lot of good to talk about it to you.

N–110. I'll be back Monday for about an hour. I enjoyed talking with you. . . . I too was in the service and some of these experiences are rough. [*Giving information. Expressing positive feelings. Accepting his right to feel as he does.*]

N–111. Good-bye, Mr. G.

P–112. Good-bye, Miss M.

Second Hour

(The patient was in the shower room when the nurse arrived. When he finished, he walked toward the nurse, smiling.)

P–1. I was wondering if you would come today. I thought you would see about getting me some heat treatment for my back. It bothered me a great deal over the week end.

N–2. Are you getting some kind of medication for it? [*Exploring.*]

P–3. No.

N–4. Did the shower help? [*Encouraging evaluation.*]

P–5. Yes.

N–6. I will ask about it when I leave to see if there is some medication that can be given. [*Offering concrete assistance.*]

P–7. Yeah.

N–8. How are things going? [*Broad opening comment. Encouraging him to take the initiative.*]

P–9. All right, except for my back.
(Pause.)

P–10. I thought we had covered everything the last time. I am surprised you want to talk with me. I thought you'd want to see someone else. [*This is interesting—contradictory to what he says above. He seems to want to know that the nurse is really concerned about him.*]

N–11. I'd like to talk with you two or three times each week for some time. I thought we could talk about you and some of the things you think about. [*Giving information about the relationship.*]

P–12. You mean about suicide and killing myself?

N–13. Yes. [*Accepting.*]

P–14. I discovered it is not easy to do. It's tough to get poison and then actually doing it. It's tough taking poison or hanging yourself—it takes too much courage—to take gas. If I had enough courage, I'd drown myself; but I don't think I have enough courage.
(Pause.)

N–15. Well, why do you think you feel this way? [*Requesting an explanation.*]

P–16. I am haunted by experiences of combat.

N–17. You said things keep flashing through your mind. [*Restating an earlier remark that is relevant.*]

P–18. Yes, seeing men die. Seeing men wounded hurt me emotionally and finally resulted in a severe case of combat fatigue.

N–19. Other people had those experiences. [*Belittling his feelings.*] Do you think they feel the way you do? [*An unrealistic question. He has no way of knowing.*]

P–20. Yes, they feel the same way, but civilian life brought them out of it. Unfortunately it didn't bring me out of it.

N–21. Do you think we could try to talk about this and work through it? [*Suggesting collaboration.*]

P–22. Yes, in time.

N–23. I'd like to help you with this. Do you think there was something you should have done while in combat? [*Offering self. Exploring.*]

P–24. No.
(Pause.)

P–25. No, now I'm manic-depressive over the wounded, but I did as good a job as I could have, so I don't feel any guilt complex.

N–26. You said something about hearing voices; have you heard them today? [*Introducing a topic from the last conversation.*]

P–27. Yes.

N–28. What did they say? [*Indicating the existence of an external source. Perhaps the nurse could just say, "Tell me about it."*]

P–29. I heard my sister's voice. She was complaining about her problem of getting along with my mother and father.

N–30. In what way? [*Offering a general lead.*]

P–31. Just trouble—grouchiness. About just getting along, that's all.

N–32. How old is your sister? Does she go to school? [*These questions could be interpreted as "probing" by the patient.*]

P–33. She works.

N–34. What does she do? [*And the nurse shifts the focus from him to his sister. Perhaps the nurse could ask, "Would you like to tell me more about these members of your family?"*]

P–35. Factory laboring work and lives at home.
(Pause.)

P–36. I heard another voice—a voice telling me to kill myself.

N–37. Tell me more. [*Exploring. Encouraging him to continue.*]

P–38. That's the one I hear more often, telling me to kill myself. I haven't slept very well the last couple of nights.

N–39. Do you hear voices at night? [*Seeking clarification.*]

P–40. Yeah.

N–41. What did they say? [*Encouraging description. Perhaps the nurse would learn more by asking for the exact words he hears: "Exactly what did you hear?"*]

P–42. Kill myself.
(Pause.)

P–43. It's not my sister's voice that tells me to kill myself; it's a man's voice. [*The nurse may want to ask, "Does the voice sound as though it comes from someone you know?"*]

N–44. How do you feel about this? [*Encouraging evaluation.*]

P–45. I agree; I want to die. If I had enough courage, I'd drown myself, but I haven't enough courage and that depresses me.

(He looked at his hands, which were cigarette-stained and shaky.)

P–46. I lost control of my hands; they are shaking involuntarily, and they pop up voluntarily. [*The nurse might want to find out if this happens often and if it is related to what he is thinking.*]

(At this point the patient seemed quite tense and restless and was moving around. Pause.)

N–47. Did you have visitors yesterday? [*Introducing an unrelated topic. The nurse could ask, "What are your thoughts now?"*]

P–48. No, I didn't expect any. I discourage visitors—it's too long a trip for them.

N–49. Where do they come from? [*Seeking clarification.*]

P–50. New York.

N–51. Have your parents visited you since you are here? [*This seems like probing. The patient should take the initiative.*]

P–52. Yes.

N–53. How do you get along with your parents? [*Probing.*]

P–54. All right.

N–55. Tell me about this. [*Exploring—but it is a subject the nurse initiated.*]

P–56. My father is a bricklayer, and my mother is a housewife. My father is 50 years old, and my mother is 45. There isn't much to say. They have a laundromat on the side. Occasionally play the horses. I have a younger brother, 14; and 2 sisters, 27 and 25. I am 29. My younger brother goes to school. The rest are all working. One sister is a housewife.

N–57. Do you all live in the same house? [*Exploring. The nurse seems to be taking a case history. Such questioning is likely to be viewed by the patient as probing.*]

P–58. We live in the same building—an apartment house.

N–59. Did you work for your father before you came here? [*Introducing another topic.*]

P–60. Yes. I worked in the laundromat before coming into the hospital.

N–61. Did you like your work? [*Encouraging evaluation. Most of this is irrelevant—at least now.*]

(The nurse lit his cigarette for him, and he moved around in the chair to a more comfortable position as though his back were painful.)

N–62. Did you hear voices while working at the laundromat? [*Probing.*]

P–63. Yes.

N–64. What did they say? [*Encouraging description. Better not to refer to "they."*]

P–65. Kill myself.

N–66. What do you think about this? [*Reflecting.*]

P–67. I agree. I tried; I stopped in the middle each time.

N–68. Is it because you think there are some things you would like to live for? [*Verbalizing what he may be implying.*]

P–69. No, I didn't have the courage.

N–70. What did you think about when you did this? [*Encouraging description.*]

P–71. I am glad when I start and disappointed when I cannot continue.

N–72. How do your parents feel about this? [*Exploring. This sounds as though the nurse is trying to make him feel guilty.*]

P–73. They are disappointed.

N–74. In what way? [*Seeking clarification.*]

P–75. Disappointed that I feel this way.

N–76. Then how does it make you feel? [*Reflecting. Encouraging guilt?*]

P–77. I don't feel any disgrace about it. Nobody else knows about this except them.

N–78. Does your sister know? [*Probing.*]

P–79. She may know. Does this report go to the doctor?

N–80. No, I discuss it with him, but the whole report doesn't go to him. [*Giving information.*]

P–81. My back is breaking; it really hurts.
(Pause.)

N–82. What are you thinking about now? [*Offering broad opening comment.*]

P–83. About my combat experiences. [*Since this is on his mind most of the time, it does not help much to talk about other things.*] About the time they got inside the patrol—the enemy. It's almost impossible what they did.

N–84. Then what happened? [*Offering general lead.*]

P–85. The sergeant took a shot at one of them and got a medal for it.

N–86. How did you feel about this? [*Encouraging evaluation. Better worded, "What were your feelings?"*]

P–87. I was horrified at the idea. See my back is breaking. [*What horrifies him exactly?*]

(He moved about cautiously and seemed quite nervous. Another patient came over to explain that he had "psychomotor activity" and had to move around from time to time. Also that he was drowsy and possibly had hypertension.)

P–88. I had a bad cold for the last couple of days.

(Another patient interrupted, talking about the effects of a new drug. Another patient came up for a light.)

P–89. My back hurts; I don't have anything more to talk about.

N–90. I'd like to come back again to talk with you. [*Offering self.*]

P–91. Yes, come again; I appreciate it.

N–92. I will be over Wednesday morning. [*Giving information about return.*]

It may be helpful for the nurse to ask him to let her know when either the auditory or visual experiences intrude into her conversation with him; then he should be asked to describe them as they are occurring.

His need to commit suicide seems more related to obeying the "voice" than to carrying out what he perceives to be his own wishes.

The nurse should try not to introduce unrelated topics—either letting him break the silences or asking him to tell her his thoughts.

Third Hour

(When the nurse arrived on the ward, she learned that the patient was to go out with the group to occupational therapy in 15 minutes.)

P–1. There is a chair (pointing to chair).

(The nurse pulled over the chair and sat down.)

N–2. What would you like to talk about today? [*Giving a broad opening.*]

P–3. I was taken off medication, and I feel better.

N–4. In what way? [*Offering a general lead. Encouraging description.*]

P–5. My hands are not popping up any more.

N–6. What else? [*Offering a general lead.*]

P–7. I feel better in general.

N–8. What does that mean? [*Seeking clarification. Better worded, "Tell me in more detail."*]

P–9. All over.

N–10. Tell me more. [*Exploring.*]

P–11. I would like to ask you a question. Did you see about getting me something for my back, heat treatment or something?

N–12. When I leave, I will see the nurse and ask her to discuss this with the doctor for you. [*Promising referral.*]

P–13. Okay.

(Pause.)

N–14. Have you been hearing voices? [*Introducing unrelated topic. Rather abrupt. If the nurse feels she must introduce the topic, she should lead up to it naturally.*]

P–15. Yes.

N–16. Would you tell me about them? [*Encouraging description of perceptions.*]

P–17. The voices keep telling me to kill myself.

N–18. Kill yourself? [*Restating.*]
(Pause.)

N–19. Was this a man's or a woman's voice? [*Exploring.*]

P–20. A man's voice.

N–21. Do you recognize the voice? [*Encouraging evaluation of perceptions.*]

P–22. No.

N–23. How do you feel about this? [*Encouraging evaluation. The nurse had an opportunity at this point to ask what the voice said.*]

P–24. I think it's a good idea. I want to kill myself; I want to commit suicide; that's how I feel about things.

N–25. You have nothing to look forward to? [*Verbalizing the implied. This was appropriate.*]

P–26. Yes, I have a younger sister to live for. [*Worth exploring this relationship.*]

N–27. This doesn't seem to hang together. You say you have a younger sister to live for; then you want to kill yourself? [*Seeking clarification. Certainly indicated.*]

P–28. I have nothing to live for—not myself. [*Worth exploring. The nurse might have restated this questioningly.*]

N–29. How about your family? [*Encouraging evaluation. This, however, takes the discussion away from the patient a bit.*]

P–30. I don't love them.

N–31. Why? [*Requesting an explanation. The nurse might say, "There's ill feeling?" or something of this sort.*]

P–32. It's because we don't get along.

N–33. Tell me more. [*Exploring.*]

P–34. About what?

N–35. About everything—do you think this is part of your problem? [*Clarifying. Reflecting.*]

P–36. Yes.

(At this point another patient came up and interrupted him, offering the nurse some raisins. She thanked him kindly, and he finally left.)

N–37. I'd like to hear more about your family problems. [*Getting him back to the topic. Exploring—to encourage more detail.*]

P–38. We quarrel all the time.

(At this time a nursing assistant called the group for occupational therapy, and the patient asked the aide if he could stay on the ward.)

P–39. You know, Monday through Friday from about 9 to 11 we go to the O.T. shop.

N–40. Well, when we discussed this last time you told me you were on the ward all day. [*Restating patient's previous comments.*]

P–41. I know; I forgot.

N–42. Then after this I'll come in the afternoon. [*Giving information.*]

P–43. Okay.

(The nurse further explained to him that when he was scheduled for an activity, it was expected that he attend and that her visits would be at a time when he was on the ward. The patient nodded.)

N–44. What do you quarrel about with your family? [*Bringing him back to the subject being discussed. Encouraging description.*]

P–45. We quarrel about everything.

N–46. What was the last thing you quarreled about? [*Focusing. Appropriate at this point.*]

P–47. I don't remember. It was something about my sister. She married a guy I don't like.

N–48. Why? [*Requesting an explanation. She might ask, "What kind of person is he?"*]

P–49. Because I feel he was worthless, and I was right; now they are getting a divorce.

N–50. How did your mother feel about this? [*Asking him to evaluate feelings of another person. Not too appropriate.*]

P–51. She had no comments to make.

(At this point they called in for occupational therapy, and the patient left with the group. The nurse told him she would visit the shop in about five minutes to see what he was doing. She visited with the ward nurse and told her about the complaint the patient had concerning his back. The ward nurse made a note and said she would discuss it with the doctor. When the nurse visited the occupational therapy shop, the patient was pacing the floor. She asked him if he had a project.)

P–52. Yes, I'm making bookends.

N–53. I'd like to see them [*Expressing interest.*]

P–54. Not now; I'm in no mood. I don't feel like working.

(He continued to pace the floor.)

N–55. I'll see you tomorrow. [*Giving information. As long as she was there and he did not feel like participating, it might have been worthwhile to try to explore his "mood"—perhaps leaving when it had altered for the better. Otherwise, he might feel that she left him—deserted him—when he was most uncomfortable.*]

The nurse should try not to introduce other people into the discussion, as she did when she asked, "How about your family?" and "How did your mother feel about this?" It may seem to him that they are more important to her than he is. Not only is he likely to be quite self-centered right now, but he may have a lot of hostility toward various family members. Other than the sister of whom he seems fond, he appears to have little positive feelings for the rest. When he brings up specific persons, she can encourage him to give more detail—but she should not push this or bring others up first.

People who want to die usually feel that no one really cares for them—they prove it to themselves by distorting or reading into what others say until they make it appear that others think only of themselves. The nurse must watch everything she says that could be misinterpreted in this manner or that seems to put others before the patient.

Fourth Hour

(When the nurse arrived on the ward, Mr. G. was in the bathroom shaving. He walked toward her.)

P–1. I will get you a chair.

N–2. You just had a shave. [*Making an observation. Giving recognition.*]

P–3. Yeah, I feel good. I had a good breakfast today, and I have been in a pleasant mood all morning. So what do you want to talk about?

N–4. About you. Anything you want to mention. [*Giving a broad opening—yet focusing on him.*]

P–5. Yes. They didn't tell me in Korea that I could get a silver star. All I needed to do was ask for it.

N–6. Why? [*Requesting an explanation.*]

P–7. For the action I had seen.

N–8. You did not ask for it? [*Seeking clarification.*]

P–9. No, I didn't.

N–10. Would you like to have a silver star? [*Reflecting. Encouraging evaluation.*]

P–11. Yes, I realize it was a mistake not putting in for it. I was very worried. What brought me to the hospital was my sister; it hurt my mental condition. My sister broke up. I wanted her to go out and associate with someone better—not exactly that, but to have a good husband. She married this guy; now she is trying to get a divorce—then she'll marry another man and get married in the church. She's got a job now, and she is saving articles for her new house.

N–12. Just exactly what about it worries you? [*Seeking clarification.*]

P–13. About the things he did [her husband]. The income tax people came and said he owed them $400 and he wasn't doing anything about it. He left her. That's what I was afraid of.

N–14. Where were they married? [*Exploring. Focusing on a minor detail.*]

P–15. In New York. I was the only one at her wedding. No one else showed up.

N–16. Who married them? [*Exploring. Again, only of minor importance.*]

P–17. They got married in his church—a Protestant church—some kind of a Protestant church.

N–18. Is she a Protestant? [*Seeking clarification.*]

P–19. No, Catholic.

N–20. Is her new boy friend a Catholic? [*Probing—or at least he could feel this way. In addition, questions that can be answered "yes" or "no" usually do not get far.*]

P–21. Yeah. My brother Jim is doing good. He is 14 now. He likes to wrestle with me, but he is getting too big. He is a tall boy.

N–22. Does he go to school? [*Probing.*]

P–23. Yes, a parochial school and having a good time.

N–24. After your sister was married, did she live at home? [*Introducing related topic. But this way the nurse is leading him.*]

P–25. No.

N–26. Did she visit home? [*Exploring.*]

P–27. Yes.

N–28. Is this the sister that argues with your mother? [*Seeking clarification.*]

P–29. No. Oh, yeah—she is the one.

N–30. What do they argue about? [*Probing.*]

P–31. Just about everything.

N–32. Does your mother like your sister's husband? [*Asking him to evaluate another person's feelings.*]

P–33. No.

N–34. These things upset you. [*Encouraging evaluation.*]

P–35. Yes. [*It is obvious that the nurse took over the discussion.*]

(He closed his eyes and appeared to be in a light sleep. The cigarette dropped out of his mouth, and this woke him up. He picked it up, and the nurse brushed the ashes off his shirt so there would be no burning of his jacket or shirt.)

P–36. She is not the sister I depend upon. It is Georgia.

N–37. Tell me about her. [*Exploring. Encouraging description.*]

P–38. She is happily married—two kids. I gave all my records and identifications to Georgia to hold.

N–39. You think a great deal of her? [*Reflecting his feelings.*]

P–40. Yes, I think a great deal of my family.

N–41. They must think a great deal of you. [*Reassuring. Not helpful. The nurse has no way of knowing.*]

P–42. I don't know about that.

N–43. Why do you say this? [*Requesting an explanation.*]

P–44. Well, my father took me to work in a brickyard, and the work was much too strenuous for a man my size, and I asked him to help me get established in another job, and he refused.

N–45. Why do you think he refused? [*Requesting an explanation.*]

P–46. Because he don't like me.

N–47. Why doesn't he like you? [*Requesting an explanation. Too many why's.*]

P–48. I don't know why he doesn't like me.

N–49. Do you like him? [*Encouraging evaluation. This doesn't give him much choice. The nurse might ask, "What are your feelings toward him?" or "What kind of person is he?"*]

P–50. Yeah.

N–51. Did you ever tell him you liked him? [*Exploring.*]

P–52. No.

N–53. Did you sit down and talk things over with your dad? [*Exploring.*]

P–54. No.

N–55. Did you ever try? [*Exploring. He may feel that the nurse is trying to make him feel guilty by implying that he should have done more.*]

P–56. Yeah, but he didn't want to talk.

N–57. Do you think he expects too much from you? [*Encouraging evaluation. A good guess.*]

P–58. Yeah, definitely too much.

N–59. What are some of the things he expects? [*Encouraging description.*]

P–60. He expects me to buy things for the house, like lamps, lampshades, or something.

N–61. He wants you to contribute? [*Restating—for clarification.*]
(The patient nodded.)

N–62. Do you pay board? [*Exploring.*]

P–63. Yes. And he asked for more.

N–64. When you were working for your father, was this in your father's business? [*Exploring.*]

P–65. Yes.

N–66. Does he manage his business? [*Exploring.*]

P–67. Now he does.

N–68. Does your back feel better today? [*Introducing new topic.*]

P–69. No, it's just as bad.
(The nurse told him that when she left the last time she spoke with the ward nurse and asked her to tell the doctor that he was asking for treatment of his back. Pause.)

N–70. Are you still hearing voices? [*Introducing unrelated topic.*]

P–71. Yes.

N–72. Whose voices? [*Seeking clarification.*]

P–73. I don't recognize the man's voice.

N–74. There are others? [*Verbalizing the implied.*]

N–75. What does the voice say? [*Encouraging description.*]

P–76. To kill myself; to commit suicide.

N–77. How often do you hear these voices? [*Exploring.*]

P–78. About three times a day.

N–79. What time of the day? [*Exploring.*]

P–80. Mornings when I get up and in the afternoon.

N–81. How do you feel about this? [*Encouraging evaluation. Better worded, "What are your feelings. . . ?"*]

P–82. I agree with him. If I could do it, I would. I can't get the necessary poison.
(He closed his eyes.)

N–83. Are you asleep? [*Seeking clarification.*]

P–84. No, but my back hurts.
(He closed his eyes again.)

N–85. Do you expect visitors this week end? [*Introducing unrelated topic.*]

P–86. No.
(Pause.)

P–87. I think I'll call and ask them to come out this Sunday. (Pause.)

N–88. I'll have to go now—I will come back on Monday. [*Giving information.*]

P–89. Okay. See you Monday. Thanks.

Every time the patient brings up wanting to commit suicide, the topic seems to be dropped abruptly. He may interpret this as disinterest on the nurse's part—disinterest in his very life!

The nurse might pursue further his comment of having "nothing to live for—not myself."

She can also express concern about his well-being—show him that she cares about his living. She can express the hope that as he comes to understand his problems better, life will be less intolerable, e.g., "I believe that you will feel differently about this as you and I talk together exploring your problems and finding solutions for some of them."

It is strange that he has not mentioned the "torturing thoughts of battle" lately. Perhaps the nurse could start a discussion by asking that he relate all the disturbing events that have occurred that morning—with details.

The nurse is taking over a bit too much—leading the discussion. By concentrating more on the present, she can avoid this. He should lead, the nurse should follow.

Fifth Hour

(The patient was sitting in a chair with his feet on a low table as the nurse walked into the dayroom. The nurse walked toward him.)

P–1. Do you want to talk with me?

N–2. Yes. [*Acknowledging that this is so.*]

P–3. Have a seat.
(He pointed to a chair that was next to him.)

N–4. Did you get a haircut? [*Introducing a topic.*]

P–5. Last week.
(He lit a cigarette off one that he was smoking.)

N–6. What would you like to talk about today? [*Giving a broad opening comment.*]

P–7. I feel like talking, but I don't know what I want to talk about.

N–8. Did you have visitors over the week end? [*Introducing a topic. Perhaps the nurse could have just waited.*]

P–9. I called my mother, and she said that they were going to visit this Wednesday. I got to call them and ask for Jello, potato salad, and cigarettes.

N–10. You're hungry? [*Seeking clarification.*]

P–11. No, I'm eating well and get finished just about the time they start to march us out. [*Is this what it's like?*]

P–12. Did you find the guy you were looking for?

N–13. Yes. He approached me the other day and asked to have someone to talk with—so I got someone to talk with him, too. [*Giving information.*]

P–14. Oh! Somebody else?

N–15. Yes. You talked with your mother? [*Getting back to the subject.*]

P–16. Yes, I asked her how she was—said everything was okay, and I heard my father call out—he said they'd be here Wednesday, rain or shine.

N–17. She was happy to hear from you? [*Asking him to evaluate his mother's reaction to him.*]

P–18. Yeah, and I felt good too. It was good to talk with her.

N–19. They seemed glad to hear from you? [*As above. This repetition may make him wonder if the nurse doubted his reply to the original question.*]

P–20. Yes, they were.

N–21. Will just your mother and father be coming to see you? [*Exploring.*]

P–22. Yeah.

N–23. How have you been sleeping? [*Introducing a new topic.*]

P–24. Good, no dreams, and I wake up and then it's morning kind of quick like.

N–25. Have you been hearing voices? [*Introducing a new topic.*]

P–26. Yesterday.

N–27. How many times? [*Exploring.*]

P–28. Two times.

N–29. What did they say? [*Encouraging description. Better not to use "they." "They" seems to indicate an external source.*]

P–30. One voice was telling me my sister's problem, and the other voice said to kill myself.

N–31. How do you feel about this? [*This would have been a good time to ask the exact words he hears. The nurse always asks this same question and gets the same reply.*]

P–32. I go along with the idea. I'd get poison. I'd like to be deceased. I tried everything and paid a lot of money to get poison.

N–33. We're here to help you—we'd like to help you feel better about yourself. [*Giving information about role of personnel.*]

P–34. So Wednesday I'll be feeling good. I'll get visitors.

N–35. Don't you think your parents are coming because they like you? [*Attempting to reassure. Not too helpful.*]

P–36. Yes, it proves something.

N–37. What does it prove to you? [*Seeking clarification.*]

P–38. It proves they love me.

N–39. Then, why do you want to hurt them? [*Requesting an explanation. The nurse seems to be blaming him for something.*]

P–40. No.

N–41. But when you hurt yourself, you hurt them. [*Moralizing. Is the nurse trying to make him feel guilty again? He may feel that she values their feelings over his.*]

(Pause.)

N–42. What are you thinking about? [*Giving a broad opening.*]

P–43. My arm—it happened three times. I was out in the cold weather, and I couldn't move my arm.

N–44. Since you're here? [*Each incident is worth exploring. Attempting to place event in time.*]

P–45. No, when I was carrying a gun in basic training. Now when I go out in cold weather, it gets numb—some doctor said it was psychosomatic. Sometimes it is a pain in the shoulder—that's where it started—then it paralyzes the whole arm. [*Perhaps this solved his problem—if he could not carry a gun, he could not kill. Perhaps now he needs to kill himself just to prove he is not a coward.*]

(Pause.)

(Coughing.) I suffered nervousness—when I was young—a schoolteacher wrote on my report card that I was strong-appearing but very nervous. And when I was—just before going into service I had a nervous breakdown, because I was operating a grocery store and business proved too much for me. And it was after that I imagined that in the center of my head there was a small room, and I imagined that it was partially filled with blood, and this blood was splashing up against the room.

N–46. What did this mean to you? [*Reflecting. Appropriate.*]

P–47. I thought something was going wrong with me and I was losing my marbles—that I was getting sick because I know there's no such thing as a room in my head.

N–48. Do you still feel this way? [*Exploring. But he already answered this question.*]

P–49. No, I don't. I don't feel there is any kind of a room in my head.

N–50. Why do you feel you're here now? [*Testing.*]

P–51. Because I'm depressed with myself—and because I made numerous attempts at suicide, and they want to study me and help me to come around to a better outlook on life.

N–52. Are you going to try to help us? [*Testing.*]

P–53. Yes, I'm trying my best to build my morale and get suicidal ideas off my mind. I should try to make friends.

N–54. Do you believe you can do this? [*Encouraging evaluation. Perhaps this is not to be encouraged—it sounds like a bunch of clichés: "building morale," "making friends," getting things "off" his mind. Understanding—not evasion—is needed.*]

P–55. Yes, but it will take time.

N–56. Did you take your medicine today? [*Introducing new topics. Is the nurse trying to tell him that if he does not think about himself and takes part in activities, his problems will go away?*]

P–57. Yes.

N–58. What did you read?

P–59. The *New York Mirror.*

N–60. Did you watch TV?

P–61. Yes, but not too closely. I once had a condition where my brain was going around like a propeller with many thoughts; now I practice relaxing.

N–62. Does this help? [*Encouraging evaluation. The nurse might ask what he does to relax.*]

P–63. Yes, it helps. Now I have flashes—it is only sometimes that I want to commit suicide—now it's only off and on.

N–64. We want to help you. [*Offering self—and others.*]

P–65. I should look at the good part of my life and look at the good times—on the good side of things.

N–66. Do you think you need to do some positive things to make you feel this way? [*Tentatively advising.*]

P–67. Yes—need to participate in activities—enjoy myself.

N–68. How do you feel about work? [*Testing.*]

P–69. I like to work—I like to work.

N–70. Do you think this could help you feel better about yourself? [*Encouraging evaluation.*]

P–71. Yes, my morale would go up. At one time my morale was so low, my face was stiff—my nerves were so overwrought. Now I don't have a stiff face any more.

N–72. What did you do in the shop today? Did you work on the book-ends? [*Introducing somewhat related topic.*]

P–73. I just pace the floor. I do a terrific amount of walking.

N–74. Do you think this is a constructive way to use your energy? [*Reflecting.*]

P–75. Yes, when I walk I—yes, but I don't think I'm contributing something.

N–76. Perhaps sometime later? [*Indicating indirectly that some understanding of his problems is needed first.*]

P–77. I improved since I first came here.

N–78. You have a cigarette on your ear. [*Making an observation.*]

P–79. I know. It's the next one. I don't usually chain-smoke, but it's so hard to get another light so I just keep smoking. If I had a match or light it would help.

N–80. The nursing assistants will give you a light whenever you want one. [*Giving information.*]

P–81. Yes, but getting out of my chair is too much trouble.

N–82. I'm glad you seem to be feeling better today. [*Expressing interest.*]

P–83. Yeah.

N–84. We want to help you. I'll be back again. [*Giving information.*]

P–85. Yes—I want to talk with you again.

N–86. Your visitors will be here Wednesday afternoon? [*Seeking clarification.*]

P–87. Yeah.

N–88. I'll see you Thursday. [*Giving information.*]

The nurse seems to be pushing two ideas—that he should think of his family and not hurt them because they love him and that keeping busy is helpful. The former is going to have to be a conclusion he draws himself. The latter is more easily said than done. When he is anxious, he will not be able to concentrate on activities. Also he should not be encouraged to avoid his problems completely—rest from them, yes, but forget them or push them out of his mind, no.

It is important for the nurse to tell him she wants to help, but it might help to be more specific about what she means by this. She might mention this in a variety of ways:

"I want to know what feelings you have—see the ways things seem to you."

"I care about your well-being, and your wanting to live."

"By knowing more about your problems, you and I can work toward solving them."

"By talking about your feelings, perhaps in time you'll come to recognize their origin."

The nurse is getting into a rut on the voices—she has often asked him these three questions: whether he is hearing them, what they say, and how he feels about it. And each time he has given the same answers. A change in approach is indicated.

Sixth Hour

(The patient was waiting by the door for the nurse. She walked toward him.)

P–1. Do you want to talk to me?

N–2. Yes. How about these two chairs?

P–3. Fine.

(The nurse and patient sat down.)

P–4. I don't know where to start.

N–5. I'll let you decide. [*Reflecting. Giving a broad opening.*]

P–6. Let's see—I can start by saying insanity runs in the family. I have an uncle and an aunt—the uncle died insane, and my aunt has been in the hospital all her life—she's insane. He was also epileptic. He died an epileptic. I don't know if that runs in the family or not. (Pause). As far as I know, there is no insanity on my mother's side, only on my father's side.

I would say that I had an unhappy youth, as a kid I was an unhappy kid. [*His early unhappiness is worth exploring later.*] I was a member of the Boy Scouts and the Sea Scouts in my youth, and once a week we would go swimming at the YMCA.

I was very popular with the girls—at one time I was going steady with three girls at the same time, but then I got involved in business with my father and it consumed all my time. [*Worth finding out some time whose idea it was that he devote all his time to the business.*] At 16 my social life ended and I got into business at 17; I was managing a grocery store. This was quite an accomplishment at this age, but I failed in 10 months. I failed—I bit off more than I could chew; then I had a nervous breakdown.

N–7. Tell me about the nervous breakdown. [*Focusing. Exploring.*]

P–8. Well, I was in the store six days a week and closed at 10 and on Sunday, several hours—then I had to do all the packing, talking with salesmen, and I had no help. It was just too much work, and I couldn't take a rest. [*Worth exploring. What was his father doing? Who said he could not rest?*]

My ears started twitching and I told you before about the square box in my head with blood splashing against it and I got tired and collapsed from overexertion.

N–9. Did you go into the hospital? [*Exploring.*]

P–10. I just rested at home and went into the Army to recuperate. I joined the Army after that.

N–11. Would you care to tell me about recuperating at home? [*Exploring.*]

P–12. I went to the movies often because as I watched a movie, it had effect and I rested. When I stayed home, it caused me to be nervous so I went to the movies.

N–13. This box and the blood, when did that go away? [*Exploring.*]

P–14. It went away after I was in the Army about a year.

N–15. What did this mean to you? [*Reflecting.*]

P–16. It meant my nervous system was getting strong again, like an illness. I don't know how a doctor would describe it, but I know it happened to me. To me it meant the brain was overworked and it was as simple as that.

N–17. You don't have this feeling any more? [*Seeking clarification.*]

P–18. No, I don't have the twitching or the box anymore.

N–19. What were you doing in the Army when this disappeared? [*Exploring.*]

P–20. I was a medical aidman—a sergeant. I became a sergeant.

N–21. You did good work to be a sergeant. [*Giving approval. The nurse has no way of knowing the quality of his work.*]

P–22. It was not so much the good work, but three other men were shot, and I replaced them and I became a sergeant. The action was thick.

N–23. Were these men killed? [*Seeking clarification.*]

P–24. Let's see, one was Brown. He got shot in two places; the others were wounded. The litter bearer was killed, but the others were sent on. I can't watch any kind of war or military pictures on TV; I start to cry. That's what I mean when I say my Army experiences haunt me.

N–25. I would like to listen to you tell about your Army experiences; that may help you. [*Exploring.*]

P–26. You want to hear about them?

N–27. Yes. [*Accepting.*]

P–28. Well, one night I was relieved of a position—relief aidman; the patrol went out and got settled in their positions, and later in the night two enemy men came in. I worked up to the position that I was in the night before, and they asked the man in the foxhole and they [enemy] had the nerve to ask us if we saw the enemy, and they went to another foxhole and asked the same thing. They asked the squad leader the same question, and he took a shot at them and wounded the enemy, and later on they gave him a medal.

N–29. How did this make you feel? [*Encouraging evaluation. Better worded, "And what were your feelings about this?"*]

P–30. I felt he was taking a very heroic chance—just like if a woman walked up to you in a nurse's uniform and actually she is not a nurse. After he shot, then everybody started shooting, and the radioman called into where I was, and I had to go out as he and the others were badly wounded, and I did all I could. One man was seriously wounded, and the one that called died—eight died. It was the most disastrous event yet. Got a match?

N–31. No; I'll get you one. [*Offering concrete assistance.*]

P–32. No, I will.

(He got up for a light from one of the nursing assistants and came right back.)

N–33. Did the enemy get killed? [*Exploring.*]

P–34. Oh yes, sure, they killed the enemy, but the fellow who took the first shot got a medal.

N–35. The fellow who got the medal was wounded, too? [*Seeking clarification.*]

P–36. Yeah. One man was captured.

P–37. The fellow who was in the foxhole with me was captured.

N–38. That was quite a situation. [*Accepting. Reflecting feelings.*]

P–39. Yes, everybody's nerves were on edge.

N–40. And you helped them. [*Reassuring.*]

P–41. Yes, we went out to get the bodies and bring them back.

N–42. They were dead? [*Seeking clarification.*]

P–43. Yes, all but two; one was seriously ill, and one was captured by the enemy—they got the upper hand and killed everybody off.

N–44. What did these men look like that you picked up? [*Exploring.*]

P–45. They were bleeding from one place or another.

N–46. How did this make you feel? [*Encouraging evaluation. Better worded, "What were your feelings at this time?"*]

P–47. It had a much more shattering experience on me than I realized. I was losing my grip on myself—as time went by. There was another time that I remember—another time we were looking for them [enemy] and they set up an ambush—it looked as though at least a dozen were firing at us, but they were firing at the trees instead of us, but in any case, we retrieved by now. I have something much worse; my worst enemy is my old man.

N–48. Old man? Whom do you mean? [*Seeking clarification. "Old man, who was this?"*]

P–49. Well, I have an old man with me, and he didn't let me sleep and that's how I got sick. So, after I got back from patrol, he worked on me, and it was my luck the litter bearer, my assistant, took more out of me than I realized. [*The "old man" was apparently the litter bearer he was referring to.*]

N–50. He was scared too? [*Seeking clarification.*]

P–51. Well, I made up my mind, when he went there, to be calm and collected. Out there we did take turns on patrol and litter bearing, so I went out on three patrols to his one. I was totally exhausted, and I called my boss to make him understand he had to go on patrol. He didn't want to do anything—the effects began to show on me. I didn't smile; I didn't want to do anything—out there. [*His "not smiling" might be explored further.*] I began to be a sad person, all I wanted to do was smoke cigarettes and drink coffee, and to this day, all I want in this world is a cigarette and a cup of coffee. After this experience I stopped thinking.

N–52. What happened to the litter bearer? [*Exploring. It might have been more appropriate to focus on him, e.g., "You stopped thinking? Tell me about this."*]

P–53. Well, he was promoted to senior litter bearer, and he bunked with me, but the senior aide came to me later and said, "You were right about him." And he got promoted, and they wanted to send the same man out to relieve me, but the platoon leader called up and said I was not to come out. He was unreliable when the chips were down. I was kept in the back so the more courageous men could go to the front lines.

N–54. Could I come back tomorrow and we shall start from here?

P–55. Yes, I would like to have you. I would like to tell you how I was as a kid, how I was a truant; how, when I was at school, I played truant instead of going to school. Oh, yes, when I was in combat, I used to shake everything from my mind. I thought if I kept these things on my mind, I would be shot. Come tomorrow.

N–56. I will.

The nurse let the patient do most of the talking this day. There seems to be a connection between the "old man" in his story and his father, who drove him (he feels) into the grocery business. Certainly the two situations are similar. Both men seem to have expected more from him than he felt he could give. He must have hated both of them for pushing him to the limit and, at the same time, hated himself for letting them down and "failing."

Seventh Hour

(When the nurse arrived on the ward, the patient was standing by the door. He walked toward her.)

P–1. You came to talk to me?

N–2. Yes.

(Another patient approached and said: "Say, how come he gets all the attention—how about talking with me—it must be pretty nice to have a nurse come and give you attention." The nurse said, "I have an appointment with Mr. G. now, but I will try to have someone talk with you, too—would you like that?" He said, "Yes" and walked away. Mr. G. stood by patiently but appeared to be listening to every word the nurse said.)

P–3. Over here are two chairs.

(Before the nurse had an opportunity to say anything, he started to talk.)

P–4. I was unhappy as a youth, and even though I did pretty well in baseball—I was pretty good—but when I got to high school, I became a bad student and cut class. I used to wait until the movies opened, then I went there instead of school. I was left back two times, and then I quit school at 16—the first year of high school.

N–5. And then? [*Offering lead. However, this seems to indicate that the nurse wants to know what happened next, rather than know more about these earlier years.*]

P–6. I went to work delivering at the meat market—errand boy. The boss made me work hard for my money. [*Was this his father or someone else?*]

N–7. How did you feel about leaving high school? [*Encouraging evaluation. "What were your feelings?"*]

P–8. I failed because I was in a bad group. [*Worth exploring.*] In grade school I did very well and graduated with a history certificate with honors.

N–9. You have the ability to do good work. [*Reassuring.*]

P–10. Yes. Yes, I have. When I got to high school, I kept company with a bad crowd—fellows who were truants. I did what they did. I cut every class—but I was still ambitious, and while not going to school I was working. As a boy I worked on week ends and evenings. I quit the meat market at 17, and I was very much weakened by this job.

N–11. Weakened? [*Restating.*]

P–12. Weakened both mentally and physically.

N–13. Would you tell me more about feeling weak mentally and physically? [*Exploring. Encouraging description.*]

P–14. Well, I was nervous and worked so fast—12 hours a day for $3—and I was very, very tired and overworked. After that, my father bought a piece of property, and on this property was a grocery store. When my father took over the grocery store, he put me in as manager.

N–15. Did this please you? [*Encouraging evaluation. Rather than suggest a particular feeling, the nurse might ask what his feelings were.*]

P–16. Well, to be in a business of this nature is a remarkable feat—but I didn't do so well. I put in 90 hours a week in the grocery store. I did discuss how I felt when I came out of the service—I was an obvious case of combat fatigue. I should have put in for compensation, but it was a fast exam, and they didn't seem to care about a man's condition. But, in any case, I didn't talk with anyone on the way home on the ship. I was in a trancelike state and stiff face. [*The "stiff face" is worthy of exploration. Perhaps it refers to feeling lifeless.*]

N–17. Would you like to tell me the thoughts you had when you were in this state? [*Encouraging description. An appropriate question.*]

P–18. I was in a state of shock. I kept thinking about combat and the men who died, and they died without any expression on their face.

N–19. They died without any expression on their face? [*Restating.*]

P–20. Yeah.

N–21. Tell me more about this. [*Exploring.*]

P–22. The majority of the men had no complaints, they had no last-minute words to request—they just died—some died in my arms.

N–23. Some died in your arms. [*Restating.*]

P–24. Yep—couple died in my arms.

N–25. How did this make you feel? [*Encouraging evaluation. "What were your feelings at this time?"*]

P–26. This brought on my condition. Well, I just went into a trancelike state of shock; it brought on my depression. I began to feel like I was dead like a ghost. [*Worth exploring.*]

N–27. You did all you could. [*Reassuring. Not helpful.*]

P–28. Yes, I did the best I could.

N–29. This was not what you expected? [*Verbalizing what seems to be implied.*]

P–30. No, it had a deep impression on me, and later on I realized I was affected by it.

N–31. After you handled these men you felt like you were in a trance-like state. [*Restating.*]

P–32. Yes, after handling the cases, I felt and acted like a zombie—not like a human being; that's how deeply I felt. I handled about 20 seriously wounded and 10 dead men—directly involved with this number. I was the medic, and 10 died before I could get to them.

P–33. Now, what information do you want?

N–34. I want to listen to the things you want to talk about. [*Giving a broad opening.*]

P–35. When I was in the Army, I was unhappy. [*Worth exploring.*] To boost my morale on Saturday and Sundays, I went to the canteen to have a big breakfast. The only thing I looked forward to was a cup of coffee and a cigarette. When I came out of the Army, I was in this trancelike state of shock.

N–36. Was this the end of your two years? [*Seeking clarification.*]

P–37. Yeah. And I went home and I used to stay up all night smoking and drinking coffee. My mind didn't revert to civilian things.

N–38. When you were smoking cigarettes, what did you think about? [*Encouraging description. Appropriate. However, he did not answer.*]

P–39. The cup of coffee had a relaxing effect on me, and when I came out of the Army, I went to many, many movies.

N–40. You were very tense? [*Verbalizing the implied.*]

P–41. Yes, I was in a condition where going to movies I tricked myself in the process of relaxing myself, but I didn't go to a military movie—it tricked me up.

N–42. You were trying to get away from your thoughts? [*Verbalizing the implied. Timely.*]

P–43. Exactly that, it was a process to get my mind off my problems. After I came out of the Army, I went into another business with my father. I went into the business of washing machines, coin-operated in apartment-house basements. As the business became a strain, I realized that my brain was very, very weakened and that I couldn't take much of a mental strain, and I realized that I had to use my back rather than my brains to make a living, because my brain was weakened. [*Worth exploring—what gave him the impression that his brain was "weak"?*] We had the business for almost a year, and I noticed that I was beginning to get nervous again, and my ears began to wiggle, so we sold the business—got that?

N–44. Yes. [*Giving information.*]

P–45. My family didn't press me for rent money or anything, so it wasn't much need for my going to work, then I relaxed at home. Then the unexpected happened. A crowd of boys and girls sat on my stoop and called out to me—I was on the floor above—they called out for me to join the crowd—they had a girl friend for me. [*The "crowd."—who were they? Did he know them?*]

N–46. They had a girl friend for you? [*Restating.*]

P–47. Yep—and, well, I didn't want to become a member of their crowd because I felt I couldn't keep up with them mentally and physically.

N–48. You couldn't keep up with them? [*Restating.*]

P–49. Yeah. But I didn't like the girl in the crowd that was to be my girl friend, so I left home and spent all the money I had saved. [*What happened?*] When I came back, I was told that the girl who was supposed to be my girl friend—she was deceased. She had an incurable heart disease.

N–50. How did you feel about this? [*Encouraging evaluation. "What were your feelings?"*]

P–51. I was very surprised, but I always considered the situation that I would never get anywhere or be at ease with the crowd—now their attitude changed, and they became abusive to me.

N–52. In what way? [*Seeking clarification and description.*]

P–53. Well, they used to sit on the stoop and pretend enemy airplanes were coming over—they were right in a way, they were guessing that I was mentally sick from the Army.

N–54. They felt you were sick? [*Restating.*]

P–55. Yeah. So I once again left home.

N–56. Would you care to tell me where you went? [*Exploring. Encouraging description.*]

P–57. Yeah, I got a room and stayed in the room—nothing much happened—ran out of money and went home. I was very, very tense. I thought the crowd would never stop bothering me. I thought that if I stepped out the door, they would see me. I was doing crazy things, dyed my hair. I went all the way to Coney Island, and no one was there but me. I kept singing and did a lot of things that were crazy.

N–58. What were your thoughts when you were doing these things? Do you remember? [*Encouraging description. "Do you remember?" is better omitted. It seems to imply low expectations of his capabilities.*]

P–59. Everything I did I thought was the right thing to do at the time, but later on I thought they were foolish and now—I thank God I can't do anything. I can't make a fool of myself, even though I want to commit suicide—I realize it's wrong, and there I'm at a standstill—I realize it's the wrong thing to commit suicide, even though I feel this way. At home, just before going into the hospital, I was so sensitive about noise that once my sister got on my nerves, and I almost choked her to death. In combat everything was quiet, and I had to have quiet at home, and my sister got noisy, and I choked her. I realized I was sick, and I realized I should be in a hospital. I was concerned with the people and myself—with the way these various people felt about me and my reputation in general. [*Worth exploring.*]

N–60. You came here for help? [*Verbalizing the implied.*]

P–61. Yeah. The strange thing about it is that the brain used to go around at a terrible pace, and now the condition is completely reversed and my mind seems to go to sleep.

N–62. Your mind seems to go to sleep? [*Restating.*]

P–63. Yeah—my mind went to sleep, and I was staring with my eyes, and I realized these were characteristics that I had trained myself to do when I was in the Army. I never rehabilitated to civilian life because I couldn't.

N–64. We'll have to continue with this next time. It's time for me to leave. [*Giving information.*]

P–65. Okay. We did okay today.

(He got up and stretched.)

P–66. It makes me feel good to talk—it helps me to get it off my chest.

(The nurse and patient walked to the door.)

N–67. I enjoy talking with you. [*Expressing interest.*]

P–68. Me, too—and I'll be thinking about things to tell you next time.

N–69. I'll be here Monday. [*Giving information.*]

P–70. Okay, but remember I'm not here in the mornings. Come in the afternoon.

N–71. I'll remember.

He is talking quite freely. This is fine now. The nurse should warn him when her time is almost up so that he will not be in the middle of something important. The nurse could use the last 10 minutes to review or to ask the patient to summarize what he has said.

Eighth Hour

(When the nurse arrived, the patient was in the shower room. He walked toward the nurse, sat down, and began talking.)

P–1. I was thinking about what I ought to mention about getting into the hospital. The crowd—the crowd of boys and girls who came over and sat on my stoop—this crowd when they began to bother me—they didn't realize what it meant to be on the other side of the fence. It's hard for them to realize what the other fellow is going through. Well, they sat on my stoop and they hinted that I was a member of their crowd. [*What did they do?*] They were called the "Cool Cats," and I was reluctant to become a member of their crowd, and the crowd knew I was in the Army, and they pretended that airplanes were coming over and things like that, so they had me cornered. I couldn't go in and out of the house without passing them by. I realized that I was no longer capable of thinking as fast as they were—my mental reflexes were slowed down—so I decided, being that I tried everything, to ask them to go away. [*All this seems quite distorted. He seems to feel that in all relationships other people expect more from him than he has to give, and that no one really understands him.*]

I went away myself for a year. Then I came back and went away for four months, and they were still on the stoop—looking to *test* me. [*Test him for what?*] So I admitted to them that I was a weakened man and there was nothing fast about me any more. But they found ways to make me angry.

N–2. They found ways to make you angry? [*Restating.*]

P–3. Well, in one way the boys were rude to a girl in the crowd, and they kept getting rude to her and said they would be rude to her until I joined the crowd. Then one day, when my brother was coming into the house, they slammed the door on his hand and hurt him. And anything I did they made me feel foolish. If I went to a bar, they would be angry because I didn't drink with them—so I was so angry I had a rifle and I was going to shoot one of them. It was then that I knew I should go into a hospital because I knew if I wouldn't, I'd shoot one of them. Is there anything that you would like me to speak about more clearly?

N–4. Talk about whatever would make you feel better. [*Giving a broad opening. However, this comment seems to imply that the nurse understands all that has been said, that there is no need to look at it more closely.*]

P–5. The girl was the daughter of a former post commander of a legion I belong to. I thought we had something in common, and it hurt me very much to see someone hurt her. Even though she was part of the scheme of things to get me over. [*The "scheme" should be explored.*] I have something that I am sorry about—I called her father and told him about this, and I was hurt very much that they were rude to her—Jane S. Then, after the incident, there was another incident. Marie P.—she was supposed to be my friend in the crowd. [*In what way were they rude?*] She died when I was away for a year. I was serious about her because her mother dated my uncle when they were kids. [*This is interesting.*] The crowd made me pretty miserable. I was as serious as they were, and there were a couple of rotten apples in the barrel, and I thought I didn't rate. I had hoped—

I worked hard all my life, and I was ill-treated, and my life was a dangerous one, so I didn't agree with associating with the crowd. I tried to reason with them, but they had a mind of their own. [*This seems contradictory.*]

N–6. What were some of the things that you didn't agree with? [*Exploring.*]

P–7. In the crowd?

N–8. Yes.

P–9. The first thing was the girl friend they had picked out for me. It is kind of hard to live a hard life, then be disappointed with the crowd you're forced to deal with. [*In what way was he "forced" to deal with them?*] They were a fast crowd—drank heavily—and I didn't have the money to keep up with them. I would have been in debt—but, then I left home for a year. I spent it. They were a rough crowd, and one incident—three boys ganged up and beat up an older man. The man had to go into the hospital for broken ribs. Things that I didn't agree with.

The girls and boys—too much jealousy—how much money they had—jobs, what kind, or they competed in drink—and because there was no significant—no lasting meaning—so, I considered it a dangerous situation. One had a car and they used to race each other—that is dangerous. These are some of the reasons and that is why I didn't join the crowd. It was a waste of time and I probably would have married the girl who died. The girl, Marie P., that never allowed me to communicate with her—but I never managed to speak to the girl alone. [*This whole story about the "crowd" does not ring true; e.g., Why would he "probably marry" a girl who seldom spoke to him? Why would a group spend so much time involving him in their activities?*]

Oh, yes, I did—I went over to talk with her in the ice-cream parlor, and she rushed over to the phone and called her girl friends, and they rushed in. And another thing, they were kind of young for me. I was 21 when I first met them, and they were 15. Then they got an older person to join them. He had an automobile. I didn't join them because I had spent a long time building up my reputation, and I didn't want to get mixed up with them. Some of the fellows were okay, but some were rotten apples.

N–10. Why did the girl call others? [*Requesting an explanation.*]

P–11. Well, they had a complicated code of their own—the girl was not supposed to gain any amount of understanding with me. The crowd wanted me to marry the girl being almost a stranger. [*Worth exploring. What gave him this impression?*]

N–12. How did you feel about this? [*Encouraging evaluation. "What were your feelings?"*]

P–13. I didn't like this because I had adopted a few resolutions, and I was determined to make a successful marriage. It was not until every effort to be successful, and the longer you know them, the girl, the better. I hardly knew the girl. I couldn't figure out their code, so I retreated. [*"Code" —what does this mean to him? A way of life?*] I figured why make a fool of myself; I just couldn't understand it.

P–14. That's enough of one subject.

P–15. I think it would be a good idea if we talked about the relationship of father and son. My father is another complicated human being with a code of his own—that I never could figure out. He put heavy responsibility on me—that was beyond me—he asked me to do the impossible at times. At 17 he put me in charge of a business—it was a grocery store. And it was beyond me—far beyond me—it was worth $6000. And he bought it when I was 15 years old. He got me started—me working on the piers. He had me working on the docks with him in the thirties. [*In the thirties, but he is only 29 now.*] He had me down there working with men over my years, and I never should have been down there. I never liked my father because of his unorthodox way of doing things—somewhat reckless way. He gambled heavily, and he wanted me to be a gambler. He enjoyed seeing me gamble at the racetracks. He detested drink, and I liked to drink. I am quite sure that I am not the type person he wanted me to be. [*This says a lot. The nurse might want to say, "This could make a person angry."*] I went into business with him two times. Both times it was the same way. He put too much responsibility on my shoulders, and I collapsed with a nervous breakdown.

N–16. Tell me the thoughts you had when you had the breakdown. [*Encouraging description.*]

P–17. When I had the nervous breakdown, my ears would wiggle, and there was a ticking in my head—and my brain used to think fast, and I was very much on the ball—my brain was well oiled.

N–18. What were some of the things that went through your mind? [*Reasking above question.*]

P–19. Well, I only had one thing on my mind; that was business. I wanted to please my father and I tried to please him but I failed. [*Again he has made a very important statement.*]

N–20. In what way did you fail? [*Seeking clarification.*]

P–21. Well, when I was in the grocery store and I collapsed with my breakdown, it looked to me like I was walking out on him, but actually I wasn't.

N–22. Did you tell him this? [*Exploring.*]

P–23. Yeah. Then there was another time—a company split—he went to work with a brick company to get me a job—so, when I quit, he quit. He was only trying to get a good job.

P–24. Then in the second business. We had 25 washing machines in apartment-house buildings. Once again, it was the same thing like everything else with my family. He put too much responsibility on my shoulder, and I had to quit. So, with my experiences with my family—too much responsibility—this is another reason why I feel so demented—mental depression. That's why I feel so downhearted. It was too much for me to take. I always wanted very much to please my father—more so than anybody else. He is a good man and works hard and deserves success, which he has—even though he has a reckless way of doing things. I was too weak, and he didn't deserve this. [*Is this how his father always made him feel?*]

N–25. You tried. [*Reassuring. Not too helpful. It implies that even when he tries, he is not good enough.*]

P–26. Yes, I tried and I failed, but that is nothing to be ashamed of. I have a complex as a result of failing. [*Worth exploring.*]

P–27. Now my mother was always good and kind to me, and we always got along affectionately. My sisters have been very helpful since I came into the hospital and shown me very much kindness.

N–28. We've talked about quite a bit today—the crowd, business, relationships between you and your father. [*Beginning to summarize.*]

P–29. What do you use this for?

N–30. When I leave, I talk with the nurse. She adds comments to the record, if there are things that are not included to date. [*This is only a partial answer. He deserves a fuller explanation.*]

P–31. Are you working for your doctorate?

N–32. No. This is nursing—psychiatric nursing. In a medical or surgical situation the nursing procedures are of a different nature. In a psychiatric unit this is the function of a psychiatric nurse. We believe we can help you by listening to you—we want to help you. [*Giving information about her role.*]

P–33. Oh, that's fine. It's easy to talk with you—it's more relaxed this way. I get a chance to talk and get it off my chest.

N–34. I must be going. [*Giving information.*]

P–35. Okay. Thanks.

N–36. I enjoyed talking with you. [*Expressing appreciation.*]

It would help if the nurse gave a fuller explanation of the notes she keeps; actually, they serve two major purposes: (1) *to review* by herself *what he has said* thus far in the relationship so that she can understand his thoughts and feelings better and (2) *to review the role she is playing in* the relationship in order to improve her ability to help him. This can be told to him.

The patient should not feel that the nurse's notes are available to others. He should be told that he may say what he wishes in what is a confidential relationship. If the nurse believes that a particular topic should be shared with other professional persons, she should tell the patient in advance of her relating it to such persons. On the other hand, if the patient wishes his doctor to have free access to the interaction notes, there is no reason why this could not be done. The nurse may also tell the patient frankly that their relationship is being supervised by a psychiatric nurse, who reviews her progress and offers guidance.

Ninth Hour

(When the nurse arrived on the ward, the patient was out on the porch walking back and forth. When he saw the nurse, he came toward her and they sat down.)

P–1. I finally did the right thing. I started writing things down. [*This may be useful. It is better that he thought of it on his own than if it had been suggested to him.*] There are some things in my life that I have always been curious about. I had three dreams that were identical. I thought that I was on top of clouds and looking down at the earth. There was a tiny opening, and I had to jump—feet first—upright, because if I folded up, I would disintegrate. If I came to earth feet first—straight up—then I would live.

N–2. What did this mean to you? [*Reflecting. Encouraging description of perceptions. Better worded, "Do you have any thoughts about your dream's significance?"*]

P–3. That's the problem. I haven't been able to figure it out. I had this dream three times—exactly alike—and I seem to wonder now if I was mentally ill then. I felt only a mentally ill person could have such complicated dreams at 8, 9, and 12 years of age.

N–4. You had these dreams at the ages of 8, 9, and 12? [*Restating.*]

P–5. Yes, they weren't dreams that a boy of my age could dream up. Another curious thing happened that made me think I was mentally ill at an early age: One night, I imagined that all the stars were crashing down on me, and I fell into a trance, and I started screaming, and my father came over to see me. I seemed to have gone out of my head.

N–6. Was this a dream? [*Seeking clarification.*]

P–7. No, it wasn't a dream. At an early age I was very popular with girls. When 13, I was going steady with three different girls—at the same time. Later on, the reason why I went to work in the grocery store and took over management was because I wanted to get married to one of the girls, Sue. [*Now he says the job was his idea. This needs clarifying.*] And

I felt to get a position and money this was my chance—a steady job and marry Sue.

P–8. My mother and father may come today. Would you like to meet them?

N–9. Yes, I would. [*Expressing interest.*]

P–10. They'll be downstairs. What happened was I failed in the grocery business, and because the business kept me so busy, I didn't have time to spend with the girl, and she married someone else. So after that I knew I would be drafted soon. I joined up to get my military service in. [*Earlier he said that he joined to "recuperate."*]

P–11. I felt bad about Sue, but not so bad that I— [*What? Worth exploring if it comes up again.*]

P–12. When I was young, I was an extreme extrovert. But resulting failures in my life and then the final military service—the period in Korea —I changed into an extreme introvert. My father used to ask me why I didn't go out and drink and have fun with fellows. [*Earlier he said that his father detested drinking.*] But when I came home from the service, I resolved to sit all alone watching TV, drinking coffee, and smoking cigarettes —and because my family didn't press me for rent money, I didn't work, and I used to sit up all night long and go to bed at dawn, which is the habit I got into in combat in Korea. Even now I can't shake the habits that I picked up in combat in Korea.

P–13. When I was 16, I wanted to become a writer, and once when I got into a company and bought a Royal typewriter for $100, I wanted to become a short-story writer.

P–14. My relative that had more influence on me than my father was my Uncle Greg. He visited us often. We went to the racetrack often—he, my father, and I. He was a longshoreman, and one day he came to the house, and I was alone. He was looking for my father to go to the racetrack with him. I noticed that he was nervous, and he dropped dead at the racetrack of coronary heart attack. We used to talk a lot together, and we were closer than my own father.

N–15. What were some of the things you talked about? [*Exploring. But what he wants to tell is what his uncle was like, and how he differed from his father.*]

P–16. He was a very well-informed man, and I especially liked to talk politics with him. It reminds me that the second most influential people were my sisters. My two sisters and I would go out of my way to do things for each other. The relative that I liked most was my Uncle Johnny or John. I've always been very much inclined to write poetry and wrote a considerable amount of it. It reminds me that I always thought I should be more close to my parents than I have been allowed. Although we went to different places together like the racetrack, etc., we still never talked together on a lot of subjects that I would have liked to talk about.

N–17. Such as? [*Offering a general lead.*]

P–18. My position in life and where I was going as an individual of society, and how I would end up in life, or in general plan about living. So, from my point of view in comparing myself with other boys, I would say that my parents were not parents enough. I should have gotten more attention in terms of teaching me about life in general.

(He looked at the paper on which he had made notes.)

P–19. My attitude toward relatives when I was quite young—I used to visit my Aunt Peggy, and once in a great while I used to visit my Uncle John, and that's my total extent of visiting relatives.

P–20. Oh! As a friend and playmate I used to pal around with my Cousin Tommy. He is my Uncle Greg's son. We more or less grew up together. When I was eight years old, we moved from Linden Avenue to Fourth Avenue and Sixteenth Street, and for the first time in my life I palled around with a crowd of boys. We called ourselves the Rams. There were about eight members in the crowd, and all of us used to dress the same way—dyed black Eisenhower jackets and blue pants. I was involved in more fights, then, than any of the rest of the boys. I used to go swimming quite often, and we used to play stickball and play touch football in the streets.

N–21. Tell me about the fights. [*Exploring.*]

P–22. Yes. In my youth I was involved in about five fights, and the first one was involved with my cousin. We were walking along Third Avenue, and two fellows just asked us quite simply to fight. So I fought one and gave him a bloody nose, and we knew that the two boys were going to go get their gang—so we ran off.

P–23. The second fight was with my Cousin Tommy. He admitted he was somewhat jealous of me, and we fought, and I won that fight also.

N–24. Did he hurt you? [*Exploring. The nurse might have asked, "Jealous of what?"*]

P–25. No, he didn't hurt me at all.

P–26. The only person who caused me friction was one tall guy who thought he was the leader of the crowd, and I was in competition with him for the leader of the crowd. I was unhappy with the crowd, and I delighted at going into business at an early age and at the process of being preoccupied. I was delighted to take care of business so that I didn't have to hang out with the crowd. Even at 13, I was more successful with girls than the average boy.

N–27. You were more successful with girls than the average boy? [*Restating.*]

P–28. I was going steady with three girls at the same time.

N–29. What do you mean by going steady? [*Seeking consensual validation.*]

P–30. By seeing a person daily and admiring that person to the exclusion of other boys and girls is what I call going steady. [*Pretty contradictory to do this with three. Nor does it sound reciprocal.*]

P–31. But at the age of 15, my family didn't give me any time for girls and from the age of 15 to the present I haven't gone steady with a girl.

N–32. How do you feel about this? [*Encouraging evaluation. "What were your feelings?"*]

P–33. I feel that everything I did in business was a waste of time. I feel that I should have married at a very young age—I was ambitious at a young age about girls. And I became revolted over what attempts I had made in business. It reminds me of what I told a friend shooting pool in a billiard parlor—I told him it was a waste of time to shoot pool when he should be trying to pursue and understand women.

P–34. Nowadays—a year ago, I came to reason that my life was going away fast, and I gave all my time to the subject of pursuing and understanding the opposite sex or girls. I decided that I did as the saying goes—turn over a new stone in my effort to reach girls—so I went to satisfy curiosity to an introductory service, and I was completely surprised and delighted with the girls I was introduced to through the introductory service. When I get out of the hospital, I intend to do nothing else except date girls from the introductory service.

P–35. At the introductory service you sign a contract for $100, and they mail a letter to you, with names, addresses, and 'phone numbers of girls. I asked them how many girls I would be introduced to for $100, and the man said to as many as 25 girls if he had to. I met five different girls, one a high-class German girl from Penn Park. She was a schoolteacher, but she was far too much out of my class to be satisfied with me, although I liked the girl. However, at this time, I was only interested in realizing if the introductory service was worth it. And I discovered that it was well worth the expense.

P–36. The second girl I liked, and I expect to go back and if I can meet this girl again—well, I seriously intend to marry her. She was a girl who had traveled extensively and came from Europe. [Patient spelled "Europe" for nurse.] All I did was to have coffee and cake with her in a small restaurant, but I didn't call her up again because all I was really doing was investigating the agency. When I go back again, it will be with a serious effort to meet and marry a girl.

N–37. We'll continue from here next time? [*Again, it might help to stop a few minutes sooner and summarize a bit, rather than terminate so abruptly.*]

P–38. Well, I'll write things down as I did this time—it's easier as I don't have to try to keep so many things in my head, and it relieves me to write and to tell you—okay?

N–39. Yes. (Giving him some paper.) I'll be over Friday. [*Giving information and something concrete.*]

The nurse is allowing the patient to take the initiative and stopping him only for purposes of clarification. This is fine for now—he obviously needs to express his thoughts. By dwelling on the past, he may be avoiding present problems, but he will come to his present difficulties in his own good time.

Tenth Hour

N–1. I found I could come today instead of tomorrow to talk with you. [*Giving information.*]

P–2. All right, I'll get my paper. I have discovered this morning that I got a book out of the library, but I just can't read books.

N–3. Do you find it difficult to concentrate? [*Verbalizing the implied.*]

P–4. Yes, I found it difficult to concentrate. When I was feeling better, I used to do a lot of reading and I loved reading. My ambitions as a youth were to be a writer, lawyer, or some sort of a brain student, like brain surgery. I felt very much relieved when I met girls through the introductory service. I had given up the idea of getting married before I went to the introductory service. But my ambitions were restored as a result of the introductory service. At the introductory service the girls were very easy to talk to and understand.

P–5. When I was in combat in the Army, I wanted to die; I wanted to get killed. [*Very much worth exploring. To let it pass seems to imply indifference.*] I volunteered for combat. As a result of combat, there were times that I could not control my hands. Once my sister got me very angry, and I choked her so long she fainted and almost choked to death, and I am sorry.

N–6. She knows you're sorry. [*The nurse is focusing on the sister's feelings rather than on his. She might better have explored what led up to the event.*]

P–7. Yes, I sent $50 to buy her a new coat when I was at K. Hospital. It was then that I discovered that I had developed a killer's instinct.

N–8. How do you feel about this? [*Encouraging evaluation. Better worded, "Tell me about this."*]

P–9. I feel a strange enjoyment at the prospect of killing someone. [*Worth exploring further. Is this "someone" anyone in particular?*]

N–10. Strange enjoyment? [*Restating. The nurse should not express undue shock at this idea.*]

P–11. Yes.

N–12. Would you explain this? [*Seeking clarification. Better worded, "Can you make this more clear?"*]

P–13. Well, as a result of my combat, I got into the habit of wanting to kill the enemy, of course. When I came home from the Army, I never managed to shake myself of Army habits.

N–14. Do you still feel this way? [*Encouraging evaluation.*]

P–15. Yes, and I realize it's wrong to want to kill, but the thought has become so ingrained, I still feel this way.

N–16. You know that it is wrong? [*Restating.*]

P–17. Yes, and I realize it's wrong. I still feel this way. For such a long time I looked forward to kill the enemy, and the habit has become so strong that I couldn't break myself of the habit.

P–18. Well, now we will talk about something more pleasant. All my life I have worried about getting married.

N–19. Worried about getting married? [*Restating.*]

P–20. My aunts—four of them were divorced, and I didn't want that to happen to me. There was one thing in life I wanted very much—a successful marriage—and as the years went by, I became frustrated with the problem.

N–21. Frustrated with the problem? [*Restating.*]

P–22. Yes, and I did give up hope of finding a girl and reaching an understanding with her and having a happy and understanding marriage, but when I went to the introductory service and after meeting a few girls, the hope of getting married became restored. I have found the girls at the introductory service very polite, honest in their conversations, and very easy to talk to.

P–23. There was a time when I wanted to kill my mother and father. I bought a rifle, but I didn't have enough nerve to shoot them. I was angry with them because my sister married a man that I didn't think was right for her. My opinion of them getting married appears to be correct because after five stormy years of marriage, they separated, and now my sister is trying to get a divorce. When this fellow Sam left my sister, some months later my sister discovered that he had run up bills that he did not pay, and three different companies tried unsuccessfully to put my sister in jail.

P–24. My youth was a fearful one. I never got the comfort I believe I should have gotten from my parents.

N–25. You have some strong feelings about this? [*Reflecting.*]

P–26. Yes, I feel the loss very much and I deeply feel the loss.

N–27. Talk more about this. [*Exploring.*]

P–28. Well, I have a father who enjoys taking risks. Perhaps he is a little mentally ill himself because my uncle and my aunt, who are his brother and sister, are both insane, so insanity runs in my father's family. As an example of the risk he took with me, he once allowed me to drive a truck up a second ramp of a pier and the truck had no brakes.

N–29. He knew this? [*Seeking clarification.*]

P–30. Yes, he knew, and I very nearly missed backing the truck off the pier.

P–31. All my life I felt the loss of a mother and father that were honest and warmly affectionate to me.

P–32. When I came home from the Army, I was still in a foxhole staring out at the night and imagining that I was still on guard against the enemy. Various habits clung to me. As an example, I would sleep all day and sit up all night as I did when I was in combat in Korea. When I came home, I became an extreme introvert and did not look forward to going out with friends. All I did was sit in my room, drinking coffee and smoking cigarettes.

P–33. My mother and father visited me yesterday and brought me cigarettes, a piece of cake, coffee, and an orange soda. [*Their bringing him things seems very important to the patient.*]

P–34. I injured my back when I was wrestling with a fellow named Robin of the Cool Cat crowd.

P–35. I injured my arm in the Army. I first remember injuring it in basic training. I first remembered a slight pain in the shoulder when carrying the rifle on guard duty in basic training. The pain got worse, and when I came out of the Army, I happened to be in a situation of being in cold weather for a few hours, and I could not move my shoulder at all. The arm became motionless when in the cold. I do a lot of painting. It has the effect of relieving my thoughts.

N–36. How did writing all the things down affect your thoughts? [*Encouraging evaluation. The nurse appears to have inadvertently changed the subject.*]

P–37. Well, it was a mental relief to write down topics of discussion because it is a strain to think of facts extemporaneously.

P–38. When I first went into the Army, I had a difficult time in basic training, and I failed to be on good terms with the sergeant in charge of us.

N–39. Would you like to tell me more about your relationship with the sergeant? [*Exploring. Appropriate. There may be a parallel here with the father-patient relationship.*]

P–40. In basic training I had considerable inability of keeping the basis of training. The result was I didn't keep up with the rest of the men.

N–41. Go on. [*Offering a general lead.*]

P–42. The sergeant's attitude would be that I wasn't working hard enough, although I was making every effort to keep up with the men.

P–43. I have run out of topics of discussion. Can you think of any?

N–44. You could talk about the things that make you feel a little better. [*Encouraging evaluation and description. However, it might be better to say ". . . the things that cause you concern." He is unlikely to know what will make him "feel better."*]

P–45. Yes, talking has somewhat relieved me. It is always a patient's desire that he or she would be understood as completely as possible by the doctor. It seems to me that any risks as a child would happen to me. I couldn't seem to avoid mischievousness and action of a sort are determined by the company one keeps.

P–46. It seems that I always came into company with the wrong kind of boy. I never seemed to enjoy anything.

N–47. Anything? [*Restating for clarification.*]

P–48. Except a few girl friends that I had. I spent most of my time with a gang called the Junior Rams, and the crowd seemed to comprise all wrongful doings. We would sneak over the fence of the city swimming pools in the summer, and once I used to do a lot of hitching on to the sanitation trucks on roller skates and let the trucks pull me. One time a truck stopped short, and I almost went under the wheel, and so I never did hitch on to any passing vehicle again with my roller skates. Once when I was five years old, I was in a big vacant lot with my Cousin Tommy, and there was a little fire there. I built it into a bigger fire and frightened my Cousin Tommy, and he ran home. It seems that life and youth were a constant proving of one's nerves. [*Very important.*]

Okay, that's enough. We did a little better today. I will have plenty to talk about next time—Monday.

The nurse might from time to time review what he is saying that seems important. They are his words, but her restatement of them (if and when the subjects come up again) might encourage him to explore them further. Such things as: "My father has a code of his own that I could never figure out. He asked me to do the impossible." "I'm not the kind of person he wanted me to be." "I wanted to please him, but I failed." "I was too weak, and he didn't deserve this." "There was a time when I wanted to kill my mother and father." "They weren't parents enough." "I have a father who enjoys taking risks." "It seems that life and youth were a constant proving of one's nerves."

Perhaps if he can review these thoughts about his relationship with his father, he will be able to realize the mixed feelings he has toward him, loving and hating him, wanting to be like him and not be like him, wanting to be close to him and yet independent of him, wanting to please him, yet feeling too much was expected of him, and the resulting mixed evaluation of himself. When the nurse feels confident enough and when the father relationship comes up again, she might want to say something like "This relationship with your father is a complex one and an important one too. I've been reviewing what you've said about the relationship, such as (give important quotes). Perhaps together you and I can try to understand this relationship better and the meaning it's had in your life, such as in your feelings about yourself as a person."

Eleventh Hour

(When the nurse arrived the patient was in the shower room. He walked toward her.)

P–1. Good afternoon, Miss M.; I will be right with you. I have the notes in my pocket, and I want to get them.

(Patient went for his notes and returned immediately.)

P–2. I thought that when I was out of the hospital I would go to the introductory service, and in the process I would get a girl and get married. I have discovered that the introductory service is the fastest process for getting married.

N–3. You seem to think it is very important to get married. [*Reflecting.*]

P–4. Yes, in my family they put a great deal of emphasis on ways one gets married. [*Worth exploring.*] My father has connection with a brick company, and I am certain that if I was married, he would give me a job there. My father afforded me little qualifications to get married.

N–5. Qualifications? [*Restating for clarification and consensual validation.*]

P–6. Well, I suppose the most important qualifications for getting married is a job or steady employment.

P–7. Also, I was not taught understanding of people, especially girls, to any reasonable extent.

N–8. What do you mean "understanding of girls"? [*Seeking consensual validation. "What do you mean" tends to sound intimidating.*]

P–9. Well, by understanding of girls I mean knowing how to act when taking a girl on a date and how to handle personalities. I think my father further handicapped me in this sense of understanding the opposite sex by not allowing me to drink.

N–10. Your father did not allow you to drink? [*Seeking clarification—of what? He already said this. The nurse might have asked, "Handicapped you?"*]

P–11. Yeah, and I have come to realize that drinking is something you have to be used to, so my attempts at meeting with people, especially girls at parties and dances, were failures.

P–12. When I was young, I would sleigh ride until my pants were frozen stiff. I loved rain because when it rained, it takes the electricity out of the air and it relaxes me. [*Takes the electricity out of the air and relaxes him?*] When I was in combat in the Army, we never had any action on rainy nights so I have come to love rain.

P–13. When I was a young boy a girl named Margie frightened me.

N–14. Frightened you? [*Restating.*]

P–15. She shooed me away, and for years afterwards whenever I heard the song about Margie, I shivered.

N–16. What were you doing when she frightened you? [*Exploring. Is it rejection he is frightened by?*]

P–17. Nothing. I was about three years of age, just capable of remembering anything.

P–18. When I was in Korea, the answer to all our problems was simply to kill the enemy. This desire continued after getting out of the Army until to date.

N–19. You still feel this way? [*Seeking clarification. But he has already said this. The nurse seems to want him to deny it.*]

P–20. Yeah, I have an attitude that is instilled in my mind to kill people that disagree with me as an answer to a problem. [*Very important. Worth exploring. Is he saying that if he kills, then he will not be destroyed because he will no longer feel inadequate?*]

P–21. I lose control of my hands sometimes because they pop up. My hands are used to acting automatically and independent of the brain.

N–22. Does it seem that something tells you to do this? [*Indicating existence of an external source. He is saying that he might not be able to control his hostile impulses.*]

P–23. Yes, it does. I sense that my eyes are wrongfully still staring for danger, even though I left combat, and I have been in this condition many years and to date.

P–24. As I review my life, I find that I have followed the food-service industry because I have done considerably more work in various types of restaurants. This is so even though the family connections are in general shipping repairs.

P–25. The desire to kill is less than it used to be. I am at the moment more disgusted with the things I did and said before coming to the hospital. One thing I did was, I went to Shelter Island at night when there was no one on the beach and started singing.

P–26. I gave my sister's collie dog away because she never took care of it. She went through a lot of trouble to get the dog back. She unsuccessfully took the people to court. She never has forgiven me for that, but she no longer mentions it because I gave her $50 when she needed it. Another thing I did was, when I was mentally sick and unattended by the hospital, I beat my sister and mother, and they got out a summons for my arrest, but neither party went to court so the case did not come up. [*These events are worth exploring if they come up again. What actually happened?*]

The hospital gives me a chance to think things out. Once, while mentally ill, I pulled a fire alarm and beat my brother, and I annoyed girls. In one case a girl sent her mother and father to visit me at my home for the purpose of making me stop bothering the girl.

P–27. I am meeting a few fellows from other hospitals here. One thing about this hospital—I enjoy the tropical fish they have in the O.T. shop, and when I go there every morning at nine o'clock, there is coffee brought to us.

P–28. I love my family, and my parents visited me last Wednesday. They brought with them a letter—a friendly letter from my sister, Mary. Mary's problems are part of the reason why I am so mentally depressed. Her husband Sam used to smash all the windows in the numerous homes they had. He quite often beat her, but now they are separated, and my sister Mary is making an effort to get a divorce. He left her with many bills. [*He is certainly jumping from topic to topic today. He may be too anxious to focus on a single topic.*]

P–29. When I was about 12 years old, me and my gang, the Junior Rams, were in Linden Avenue in snowy weather riding our sleds, so I couldn't get anybody to ride with me on my sled down this hill called Suicide Hill. Finally I got someone to ride with me down the hill, and we hit upon a small mound of ice, and I busted one of my front teeth off. Since then I got a cap put on the broken tooth by a dentist.

P–30. Since I have been in the hospitals, I have gotten into two fights, both in other hospitals.

P–31. I love my breakfast more than the other meals, especially when there are bananas.

P–32. I have written letters to my sister and brother that I want each of them to hold $500, and if they need to, they can spend it. Another thing I did when I was sick and unrestrained was I spent all my savings.

N–33. What did you spend the savings for? [*Exploring.*]

P–34. I bought and sold three cars and much clothing, discarding the clothing for no reason at all. I went drinking and went on a sort of tour with a friend that I had known in my youth.

P–35. Wait a minute; there is the contact man, and I need to see him. (He left for about three minutes and returned.)

P–36. Of the three hospitals before mentioned, I prefer this one. I like being here because we can smoke cigarettes when eating.

P–37. The voices I have been hearing lately have been sounds by men. I started hearing voices about two years ago. [*The nurse had an opening here to get more detail on the "voices."*]

P–38. I went to one baseball game in my life. It was the game between the New York Giants and the Philadelphia Athletics. A fellow took me; the Philadelphia team beat the Giants in both games. There was a double-header. My friend was so disappointed that he did not eat any of the fruit and sandwiches he had brought to the game; so although I was too young to understand the game, nevertheless I enjoyed eating the splendid lunch.

P–39. I went to neighborhood movies, and that was the extent of my doings in the world away from home. [*Worth exploring more fully. Was he prevented from doing more? If so, by whom?*]

N–40. It is about time for me to be going. You look much more relaxed today. [*Giving information. Making an observation.*]

P–41. Yes, I am—talking with you and having someone believe in me makes me feel better.

N–42. Would you like some more paper? [*Offering something concrete.*]

P–43. Yes.

N–44. Would you give some thought to writing everything about voices you hear, exactly what they say and how often you hear them? [*Encouraging description of perceptions. But this might have been more appropriately timed—as when he mentioned the voices a few minutes earlier.*]

P–45. Okay.

He is bringing up a lot of minor events that seem unconnected. If this continues, the nurse may have to focus on what seems important, so that he does not just jump from topic to topic. He wants to tell the nurse all the things he has made notes on, but if what he brings up seems insignificant (e.g., "I like my breakfast more than other meals, especially when there are bananas"), the nurse might ask him what led him to bring it up or what significance it has to him.

Twelfth Hour

(The patient was on the porch, and when he saw the nurse, he looked for the notes he had in his pocket and came toward her.)

N–1. What have we decided to talk about today? [*Giving a broad opening. The plural should not be used when it does not apply.*]

P–2. We were going to talk about feelings. It reminds me of the time when I was choking my sister. [*The events leading up to the incident with his sister are worth exploring.*] When I did it, it seemed to me that I was back in Korea and shooting the enemy. I felt a certain sense of enjoyment. It apparently happened that from learning to kill in the Army that now I am sort of a pathological killer.

I don't like Western movies. Perhaps the reason is because they carry guns, and I don't like anything that involves guns.

N–3. Then you really didn't like to kill? [*Verbalizing the implied.*]

P–4. I instinctly try to choke with my hands. I think that you already know that when I watch pictures, I crack up.

N–5. You "crack up"? [*Restating for clarification.*]

P–6. Yes. That means have a nervous breakdown, and I have to walk away from the movie. Pictures that I do like are *Gone with the Wind*—serious pictures. Nor do I like musical comedies. I like pictures that are dramatic.

P–7. I made many efforts to get a high-school diploma. I studied courses in the Army, and I attended a private school. I paid money to this private school. The school was with the Lamb's Business School, and I studied shorthand. However, I never got a high-school diploma.

(The nurse told him about the opportunities to study for a high-school diploma in the educational therapy department. He seemed to know about this.) [*Giving information.*]

P–8. I am interested in the courses—as soon as I get out of this ward. But now I feel that I can't concentrate. I can't read, so that I will have to look into this when I feel better.

P–9. My father and I almost went into a business together at the Shelter Island. It was a type of game business. You could toss pennies, and if the pennies landed on the buzzer, you would win a prize. But instead of going into that business, we went into the washing-machine business. We bought about 25 machines from a very wealthy man. The route was situated in New York. The best machine locations you can get are in the housing-project buildings. I figure that a good operator could make about $25 an hour on the project machines. In private apartment houses you can make about $15 an hour, but we were making $6 an hour.

P–10. When I was in high school, my mother always gave me 30 cents a day, and I found it very thrilling to avoid school by playing hooky. [*Worth exploring. What did it seem to prove?*] I palled around with a fellow named Ram. I never enjoyed myself so much in all my life. There was a cake shop which had a cookie that I happened to like very much; so in the morning we would sign in at the prefect, and then I would cut every class. In the morning we would go to the coffee shop, and in the afternoon we would go to a movie. A fellow named Riley, who was one of the Ram's gang, also cut a lot of classes with me, and we would go to the movies together.

P–11. When I was about 11 years old, I liked a girl in the classroom. I used to stare at her, and the girl seemed to take a liking to me. One of my girl friends, upon hearing that I would do anything for her, asked me to cut off my right arm, which I certainly wouldn't do. I couldn't do that. This was the first of two occasions that I was not able to comply with girls. [*The other?*]

P–12. My mother went to the main office where all my papers are. She told me that they were going to make back payments of my disability checks, and that it would come to a little over $1000. Because I was worried about my sister Mary's financial affairs, I had asked her to hold $500 for me, and if she needed it, she might spend it on herself. I made the same arrangements with my brother Jim.

P–13. One of the happiest, and perhaps the happiest, moment of my life was when my father used to take us driving in his automobile all day and throughout the evening until my sister and I fell asleep. We used to start out by going to a factory where they sold pies for five cents each, and we would buy about a dozen. Once when I was about 15, my father took me to the wrestling matches.

P–14. When I first went to school, my mother didn't come to school to meet me, so I had to walk home all alone. [*This is surprising. Perhaps he will talk, later, more about his mother. He has said very little so far.*] I had only one thing that I could remember about the route home, and that was that I had to pass a gas station. I started walking and saw a gas station, so I thought I was going the right way, but then I saw a whole string of gas stations, and I realized that I was going the wrong way. This upset me because I was lost, and it was the first time in my life that my mother disappointed me.

P–15. I used to study very hard for a couple of months, and then for a couple of months I studied only a little. I used to go into slumps with my education. The last term of elementary school I behaved as usual. The first couple of months I worked hard, and the last couple of months I did little or nothing. The teacher graduated me with an 83 average, but she told me privately that she was giving me my mark for that part of the term when I studied and not for the part of the term when I did not study.

(He started looking over the notes on the papers he had and hesitated for a moment.)

N–16. Last time we decided that we would talk about the voices. [*Introducing unrelated topic. "We" decided? He may resent the way she put it. The nurse might ask, "Have you made any notes on the voices?" if she feels she must bring this topic into the conversation.*]

P–17. Well, I didn't hear any voices for a couple of days. Sometimes when I watch television, I would listen to a particular song, and then I can't get it out of my mind. I imagine that the song is being played over and over again in my mind. Some things, like musical recordings, seem to stick with me. A couple of days ago I got to hearing a man singing a song that's quite popular on the morning bandstand TV.

P–18. It was about a week ago that I last heard the voices telling me to kill myself. I still feel the same way about dying. I still feel that if I was let loose from the hospital, I would go to Shelter Island and try to drown myself. [*Why might he select this particular spot?*]

P–19. When I was three years old, I had a very bad fall down a flight of stairs.

P–20. I don't like staying in the hospital with a group of sick men. They do disgusting things—like spitting on the floor, picking their noses, cough, and so on. When I was here before, they made me so sick I vomited, and then I went to 15-B North.

P–21. I feel many times better these last couple of days because of an arrangement I made with my sister and brother giving them money if they need it. [*Is he trying to buy their love?*] If they need it, they have got it. Once my sister needed money, and I couldn't give her money in time, but now if she needs it, she's got it.

(Another patient walked toward the patient and nurse.)

P–22. Here's a candidate for you—Tommy de P. He would like to be interviewed.

P–23. Do you know Mr. George J.?

N–24. Who is he? [*Seeking clarification.*]

P–25. He is a night aide. He knows you. He is the best aide here.

N–26 Why do you say this? [*Requesting an explanation. Better phrased, "In what way?"*]

P–27. He is extremely sympathetic to the extent that he makes me very comfortable.

P–28. I have been in three or four hospitals, and I have come to like this one best, except for the fact that in other hospitals you can smoke in the dining room. I very much miss having coffee when I want it, and living close with a group of men nauseates me. As a young fellow, I belonged to the Boy Scouts and to the Sea Scouts Naval Cadets.

P–29. I love the porch on the wards. They are great places for reminiscing, but some of the men spit on it.

N–30. It is time for me to go. [*Giving information.*]

P–31. Okay. When are you coming again?

N–32 I will see you tomorrow. [*Giving information.*]
(The patient went to join a remotivation group.)

Since he has not been bothered by the "voices" telling him to kill himself for a week now, perhaps it would be better for the nurse not to mention them first but to let him bring them up if he chooses.

It is interesting that he is now able to direct more of his hostility outward toward his family—and less toward himself—even if indirectly by acknowledging his wanting to kill them and his "attacks" on them, real or imagined.

Perhaps the nurse will want to read his clinical record now. If she does, she should be careful not to introduce any of the history into her conversations with him. Also, if she has an opportunity to meet any of the family, she should do so. The ward personnel may be able to tell her something about how the family interacts during visiting hours. These things will give her better perspective.

Thirteenth Hour

P–1. I was invited to join a crowd, but I didn't want to be a member of the crowd.

N–2. When was this? [*Placing event in time.*]

P–3. About three years ago. They were a nasty bunch and vicious crowd of boys and girls that were younger than I was and would have amounted to a decline of my character if I joined. They called themselves the Cool Cats. There was a girl in the crowd by the name of Jane S., and as I studied the meanings of the members of the crowd, I realized the influences that brought us together—although I did nothing to show that I was willing to be a member of the crowd, I considered them, and in my qualifying opinion I thought that this girl, Jane S., was the girl in the crowd that I rated as should be my girl. [*He keeps telling the same story but with variations. It would be interesting to explore the extent to which he had actual contact with this girl—whether he ever spoke to her, for instance.*]

That's the way it was with the crowd. The boys and the girls sort of paired off as boy friend and girl friend. I wrote her a couple of letters to explain to her that I realized that she rated as being my girl in the crowd. She got angry and personally returned the letters. But now she had told all the members of the crowd that I considered her my girl friend. And I imagine that they were being rude to her in an effort to force me to become part of the crowd. One thing they did was throw her in the snow and kick snow all over her. I wrote her another letter; she didn't return it, but she sent me a note stating that I was bothering her and that if I continued to bother her, she would go to the severest extreme to get me to stop. What she meant was she would have me beaten up.

N–4. By whom? [*Exploring.*]

P–5. I'll come to that—one of the Cool Cat crowd of boys. I went to a party quite accidentally and danced with all her girl friends. She was a complicated girl—one minute she seemed to draw you into her friendship and the next minute doing something to hurt you. At the party she seemed hurt because I danced with everybody except her, and she started crying, and then as the party progressed, she got a fellow to take me outside in the street, and I talked myself out of a beating. I made four recordings for her.

N–6. Recordings? [*Restating for clarification.*]

P–7. Recordings—songs—and she played them at a party in an effort to make a fool out of me.

N–8. How did you feel about this? [*Encouraging evaluation. "What were your feelings?" The nurse might also have questioned his impression of her intention and its origin.*]

P–9. My feelings were very hurt because she wouldn't listen to reason. So soon after that I went into the hospital, and days later my sister told me that a fellow was looking for me at the house. There is no doubt that he was going to start an argument with me about my communicating with the girl. She didn't want to be bothered. But I was going crazy thinking that they were being rude to her because of me. [*What gave him the impression that the "rudeness" was "because of" him?*] Later on I heard from my sister that Jane S. was asking for me. I wrote her two more letters.

P–10. Another thing I did, when I thought they were being rude to her because of me, was to call up her father and tell him the whole story. This was a mistake on my part. I have just mailed a letter to her a couple of days ago.

N–11. Since you're here? [*Seeking clarification. Placing event in time.*]

P–12. Yes—apologizing for calling her father about this problem that I imagined.

N–13. Imagined? [*Restating for clarification.*]

P–14. I imagined all this—none of it was true. I also sent her a Valentines's Day card, but I didn't put my name on it. [*What events led him to this conclusion?*]

P–15. I temporarily left home, and I got a variety of jobs and quit them because I couldn't concentrate. [*What led up to his leaving home is worth exploring more in detail.*] One of the jobs I got was with a nightclub, hat-and-coat-checking service. The job wasn't the type of job one would take for making money. The pay was only $6 a night, and a reasonable meal costs $1. I met a few of the Hollywood movie stars there. I worked in three nightclubs. After I finished working, and I found myself working a 14-hour day, some of the boys and girls would go to Rector's for a breakfast. In the Copa' I handled Frank Costello's coat and Robert Taylor's coat and many others.

P–16. When I was in the Army at Camp Cooke, I finally got a weekend pass. And for the first and only time in my life I took a hotel room and enjoyed luxuries I couldn't afford, like having breakfast sent up [in bed]. Then I went to the racetrack in Mexico. I traveled by bus. I was homesick and figured that I could cure my homesickness by going to the racetrack.

P–17. On another pass I went with three other fellows to Santa Barbara in California. We went to a roller-skating rink. And I fell down a few times on the roller skates. I met a nice girl. She, her mother, father, and little brother were touring the States. Her younger brother was a champion roller skater. I gave her my address, and she wrote me a letter from Salt Lake City. Later on, as the evening progressed, we four soldiers left the roller-skating rink and started looking for the USO center. While we were walking, a short fellow of a soldier came up to us and told us that he had been beaten up by three marines. He asked us for help, so we all went looking for the three marines. We went to a place for servicemen to sleep and read and rest—quite different from the USO. We didn't find the three marines. I had a difficult time in basic training. During those first eight weeks, I went from Camp Roberts [California] to Camp Cook for advanced basic training, and it was during the first eight weeks that I imagined the sergeant of our barracks disliked me.

N–18. You imagined this, but he really didn't dislike you. [*Restating.*]

P–19. I imagined this; he was all right. I couldn't keep up with the orders that were given us, such as keeping our equipment in good condition. I was extremely tense, and then one day when we were qualifying for the M-1 rifle, I couldn't shoot the rifle.

N–20. Tell me about it. [*Exploring. Encouraging description of perceptions.*]

P–21. Yes. I started crying, but there was something that told me not to fire.

N–22. You heard a voice? [*Seeking clarification. The nurse should not jump to conclusions. She might just ask, "Something?"*]

P–23. No—no.

N–24. Just intuition? [*Suggesting possible explanation. Worth exploring further his feelings at that moment.*]

P–25. Yes, just intuition. My intuition was correct, because when this strict first sergeant gave the orders, he neglected to give the last order of the command.

N–26. What was this? [*Seeking clarification.*]

P–27. One must say "Fire" when giving a command to fire a rifle. The company commander came over to me and talked to me a few moments and pacified me.

N–28. What did he say? [*Could this be why he ended up in the medics? Encouraging description.*]

P–29. Don't remember his words. Then I told him the first sergeant did not give the order in the only way one can give the order; he didn't say "Fire."

P–30. He agreed with me—the commanding officer agreed with me that I was right in not firing the weapon. This meant that all the men that fired were wrong, and everybody else fired, but I didn't, and the idea of everybody else being wrong and my being right was the reason that I cried. It hurt my feelings because I was right and the rest were wrong. [*"Hurt his feelings" in what way?*]

P–31. I had learned in basic training that everything had to be right, and I tried to be obedient to the extent that I was tense. I was hurt because —and felt that I should follow the command.

P–32. When I was in Japan, I studied to be a medical aidman in a large building that was formerly the Japanese Naval Academy equivalent to the United States School of Naval Studies at Annapolis. They were extremely highly qualified; they had as one of their final tests to swim a stretch of water. In this final test they lost an average of 8 out of 100 men by drowning of the graduating class. [*This would seem most unlikely.*] Before I came to the hospital and when I was sick, one of the biggest mistakes I made was the changing of my name from C. to G. It cost me $75. [*Worth exploring.*]

P–33. The first presents we kids—my sisters and I—gave my mother were some pictures of flowers that my father gave us to give her.

P–34. There was a girl named Pat B., and I sort of went steady with her for three years when I was 11, 12, and 13. She had a girl friend named Hartwell. This girl, Pat, came to love me very, very much. My mother knows a Mrs. C., and she knows this girl's mother, and Pat's mother told Mrs. C., and Mrs. C. told my mother and I that Pat did a lot of crying over me. We did a lot of swimming together in city pools.

P–35. When I try to think spontaneously, I get very tense and write topics down.

P–36. How much time do we have?

N–37. It's soon time to stop. [*Giving information. He is expressing his need to know in advance that she will be leaving soon.*]

P–38. Let's quit.

N–39. Okay. [*Complying.*]

N–40. You haven't been hearing voices? [*Introducing an unrelated topic—and at a poor time. If he were hearing them, the nurse would not have time to handle the anxiety she might have created in mentioning them.*]

P–41. No.

He seems to exaggerate his success with girls and perhaps also his failures in relationships with men—which may reflect his original feelings toward his parents, an affectionate(?) mother and a father whose expectations he could not meet.

Now that he is bringing the same things up again and again, the nurse might begin to explore some of these things more fully—especially the happenings that are obviously distorted or misinterpreted. When he says things the nurse finds it hard to believe, she might ask him to describe how he came to these conclusions or came to have these impressions—especially when they relate to how other people felt toward him, such as the sergeant's disliking him or the 11-year-old's loving him "very, very much."

The nurse does not need to overdo this; she can choose what she thinks are the opportune times for this and not press if he does not give what she wants or expects. She can also express doubt now and then when he says something quite distorted, e.g., "That's hard to believe," or "How strange! Is that really how it happened?"

She may find it helpful to read back over all her interaction notes now and then and make notes from them of important statements he has made. This will make them more available to her; otherwise, it is easy to forget them and never make further use of them.

The nurse should not bring up any of his thoughts of suicide unless he initiates such discussion. Nor should she mention the voices first. He knows she is interested in them now; it is up to him to mention when and if they reoccur. To ask too often exaggerates their importance—as though the nurse is interested only in his pathology.

Fourteenth Hour

(The nurse was a little late arriving on the ward for the appointment.)

P–1. I thought this was only for two weeks.

N–2. No, in the beginning I said we would talk two or three times each week. [*Clarifying.*]

N–3. How have you been feeling? [*Giving a broad opening. "What have your feelings been?"*]

P–4. All right; feeling good.

N–5. Is there anything you would like to talk about today? [*Broad opening.*]

P–6. No, not particularly.
(There was a long pause.)

P–7. I was expecting visitors for the week end and did not get them, so I am a little upset. I called home two times, and they said they could not come because my brother-in-law broke his glasses and could not see to drive.

N–8. You talked with your mother? [*Seeking clarification. Perhaps the nurse could have focused on his feelings, e.g., "This disappointed you."*]

P–9. Yes. With my mother and my sister.

P–10. I thought we'd be through in two weeks.

N–11. Well, I do like to see you two or three times each week. [*Expressing interest. This might seem to him to be meeting the nurse's needs, rather than his. Perhaps she could just say, "You feel you have nothing to talk about?"*]

(A patient came over and said: "Aren't you going to talk to Miss M.? I am jealous. Mrs. K. comes to see me only once a week.")

P–12. I don't know what to say.

N–13. We can just sit for awhile. We don't have to talk all the time. [*Giving information about the relationship.*]

(The patient nodded and coughed and seemed quite restless. The other patient interrupted again and said: "Seconal—what do you know about Seconal?"

Nurse: Well, it's a pill to help you sleep.

Patient 2: What would an overdose do?

Nurse: It would cause ill effects.

And he walked away.)

P–14. If you would like to talk with somebody else, that's okay with me. [*It is important to handle interruptions briefly like this without rejecting the other patient, yet not getting involved.*]

N–15. No, I wish to spend this time with you. I'll just sit here. [*Offering self. Most appropriate.*]

(At the end of the hour.)

N–16. I'll be going now. I'll be back as I'd like to continue. [*Giving information. Offering self.*]

P–17. Well, you see I'm upset. I'm upset at the way they are handling my money. I asked the social worker to have a lawyer handle my money, and this was turned down. He said that the check was going to my mother, and she told me she was putting the money in her account, and I don't like this.

N–18. Perhaps when the contact man comes in, you could discuss this with him. He may be able to give you the information you are seeking. [*Tentatively suggesting course of action.*]

P–19. That's a good idea.

P–20. I'm depressed today. I don't feel like talking.

N–21. See you on Wednesday. [*Giving information. It might have helped to have said, "It's difficult to talk when you feel depressed," or something similarly accepting.*]

It would not seem that the patient was rejecting the nurse personally. She appropriately pointed out her interest in him and in continuing the relationship. She accepted his silence. This seemed to be meaningful to him because he finally expressed some of the things that were bothering him.

If he continues to bring up his expectation that the relationship was to be over in two weeks, the nurse would do well to explore this more fully—

what his feelings are about continuing, the purpose of the relationship, his role, and so forth. Even if he does not, she might want to tell him more about the purpose—giving him an opportunity to identify and explore his problems in living with others.

If he continues to feel depressed and to be noncommunicative, she can point out that she is interested in him, in his well-being and comfort, not just in what he has to say, that when he does not feel like talking, she would like to stay unless it makes him uncomfortable, and that when he can express his feelings, she will listen.

Fifteenth Hour

(The patient was stretched out on two chairs smoking when the nurse arrived. She walked toward him, and he said "Hi," smiled, and pointed to a chair next to him.)

N–1. Hello. [*Offering recognition.*]

P–2. How are you?

N–3. Fine. You're all cleaned up. [*Making an observation. Giving recognition.*]

P–4. Yes, I took a shower. The cuff on my shirt has no button.

N–5. Would you like to tell me how you're feeling today? [*Encouraging evaluation and description. Better worded, ". . . tell me what your feelings are today?"*]

P–6. Yes, I'm feeling all right; I'm looking forward to a visit from my sister. She's coming on Sunday. So I'm feeling a little better.

(Pause.)

N–7. Did you write any notes? [*Introducing a topic.*]

P–8. No, I didn't feel like it.

N–9. You aren't feeling so well? [*Verbalizing the implied.*]

P–10. I am feeling better; a little depressed, but I'm feeling better because my sister is going to visit me on Sunday.

N–11. Would you like to talk about it? [*Rather than give him a choice, she might say, "Tell me about these feelings."*]

P–12. I just did—mentally I feel depressed.

N–13. Did it make you angry because your family didn't visit you last Sunday? [*Encouraging evaluation. Better worded, "What were your feelings when . . . ?" or "Is this similar to your feelings last Sunday when . . . ?"*]

(Another patient approached and said: "It's rude to be so comfortable in front of a lady.")

P–14. She knows about my back.

N–15. I can accept it. [*Accepting. Rather vague. What is nurse accepting—his "rudeness," his comfortable position, or his back pain?*]

(The other patient walked away. Pause. Another patient came for a cigarette light, said "Thanks," and left.)

P–16. He's being interviewed, isn't he?

N–17. Yes, Mrs. K. comes to talk with him. She is with us two days a week and visits him weekly. What have you been thinking about? [*Giving information. Offering a broad opening.*]

P–18. About my sister visiting me Sunday. She doesn't have to rent a limousine—hope she can get a ride.

(He was sticking his tongue out and smacking his lips.)

N–19. Does your tongue bother you? [*Encouraging evaluation.*]

P–20. Yes, it's dry, and I have a sour taste in my mouth. They changed my medicine, and it's the new medicine.

N–21. Do you know what you're taking? [*Exploring.*]

P–22. No, two different kinds of pills.

(The personnel brought in some liquid nourishment.)

N–23. Shall I get you some? [*Offering to do something concrete for the patient.*]

P–24. No, no thanks.

(He got up and came back with a cupful. Pause.)

N–25. Has your sister been here to visit you before? [*Reintroducing previous topic.*]

P–26. Yes.

N–27. She'll be pleased to see you looking better. [*Reassuring. But the nurse has no way of knowing* her *feelings.*]

(Pause.)

N–28. Do you think you're better since you're here? [*Reflecting. Encouraging evaluation.*]

P–29. Yes, I gained about 15 pounds—but I'm not ready to face the outside world yet. I still imagine—when I hear things, it repeats over and over in my mind—keeps repeating—then something distracts me; then it changes like if I hear a song—the words linger in my mind until I have a distraction.

N–30. Is anything that I say repeated? [*Exploring. Perhaps the nurse might have asked, "What are some of the things that repeat themselves?" Surely, it is more than songs.*]

P–31. No, I don't think so—can't remember it. If it's something I like, it's repeated and strong enough for me to care. Then it sticks in my mind. [*Worth exploring further.*]

P–32. It's annoying in the O.T. shop—can't concentrate—so I pace—then I lose my strength after about 12 o'clock—then my legs are out of energy. That's why I like the morning time—the afternoons and nights I don't care for.

P–33. There's a girl I can't seem to get out of my mind and my whole system, Jane S. She made a lot of trouble for me on the outside—but I can't get her off my mind. I tried to explain something to her, and she refused to listen to me.

N–34. Tried to explain something to her? [*Restating.*]

P–35. Yes.

(Then he went into a dissertation on food and why he likes breakfast best—it is more like his mother's cooking—the rest of the meals have fancy foods. His mother's stew has only meat and potatoes in it and not other things such as onions and carrots.)

P–36. You come Monday, Wednesday, and Friday?

N–37. Yes, and if I can't come on Friday, I come Thursdays. [*Giving information.*]

P–38. Okay.

N–39. It's time to go. See you Friday. [*Giving information.*]

P–40. So long.

Sixteenth Hour

P–1. I would have written more notes, but I didn't have a pencil. I wrote some notes.

N–2. Good. [*Giving approval. Better to just be accepting.*]

P–3. I wanted to mention that these interviews have a wrong effect on me, because I talk about things that I want to forget. I was going to suggest that we cut down from three to two a week, because I am feeling a little stiff-faced, grouchy, and I'm not sleeping well—I am having dreams.

N–4. Would you tell me what you dream about? [*Encouraging description.*]

P–5. I dreamt about my Uncle Ed and my sister.

N–6. Go on. [*Offering general lead.*]

P–7. Don't remember about my sister. I was reminded of the time I went looking for a job, and my Uncle Ed told me to come back the next day and he'd put me to work. That is considered an unhappy dream—going to my Uncle Ed's is one of the crazy things I did when I was on the outside.

N–8. Tell me more. I'd like to hear what you mean by this. [*Exploring. Encouraging description. The use of "mean" tends to be intimidating.*]

P–9. To put my uncle in an uncomfortable position of giving me a job—he's a longshoreman and boss on the job, and we *never ask for favors* like jobs in our family. [*Worth exploring. What gives him the impression it is "wrong" to ask for help? What does it imply—weakness? In what way? Who gave him this impression? This would probably lead back to the relationship with his father.*] The more I think of the crazy things I did, the more I become depressed.

P–10. It's like doing something wrong. It's a sense of pride. I called him at the docks, and it's something I'm very much ashamed of. It strikes me as being a nightmare.

P–11. Before the interviews I wanted to die. Now I keep thinking I want to kill myself. What I did revolts me—I haven't got enough nerve to tell you about the wrong things I did.

N–12. I'm a professional person, and I'm here to listen to the things you choose to tell me. They will be part of your chart. I make summaries and add them to the nurse's notes. This opportunity is whatever you make of it. I'm here to listen and to help. [*Giving information about her role. Perhaps the patient would prefer that the nurse keep some things confidential.*]

P–13. There are some things on this paper that I have scratched out; it's that bad. I tell you good things, and once in a while I tell you one of the bad things.

N–14. I'm here to listen to those things you wish to tell me. [*Giving information about nurse's role.*]

P–15. I'm very worried about my sister, but she is coming along quite well. She's getting married again, and the only delay is they are looking for an apartment. I've been thinking about my vocation in life, and I was thinking that I'd make a good gardener. When I was much younger, I raised corn and tomatoes. I seemed to enjoy the work so much that it didn't seem like work. I still haven't got the patience to work at a job in the O.T. or C.T. shop as my right arm seems heavier—there is still a slight pain in the shoulder.

P–16. On three different occasions in cold weather I lost complete movement or power of the right arm. [*The three occasions are worth exploring.*] When I was a little boy, I used to buy baby chicks and raise them. I reminisce about this when I feed the pigeons off the porch. I like to travel on highways and always wanted to take a long trip on the Greyhound Bus

Lines. When I was quite young, my father used to fly pigeons off the roof-top. I've always wanted to do the same. I always liked pets and have owned three different dogs.

P–17. When I was quite young, my family used to go to a certain place where pies were then five cents each, and we would drive the car all day and most of the night until we fell asleep.

P–18. Is the time up?

N–19. Yes. [*Acknowledging that this is so.*]

P–20. Well, I'll see you Monday—I need some paper.

(The nurse gave him several sheets of paper, and he walked to the door with the nurse. He said he would see her Monday and was looking forward to seeing his sister on Sunday.)

Not too much is happening, but one comment was most worthwhile, i.e., the one about telling the nurse one of the "bad" things once in awhile. She was accepting and encouraged him to continue expressing himself as much as he is able.

Seventeenth Hour

(The patient was pacing in the hall on the nurse's arrival. He exchanged greetings; he said he had made some notes. He stated that he had no visitors over the week end but that he talked with his family on the telephone and that his sister was coming by limousine on Wednesday. He did not appear depressed at not having visitors, as he did previously. The patient and nurse got settled on the porch.)

P–1. Is there anything in particular that you wanted me to elaborate on?

N–2. At this time whatever you wish to talk about. [*Giving a broad opening. Perhaps he is indicating his readiness to look more closely at the events and feelings he is describing.*]

P–3. I always feel better when it rains. In Korea whenever it rained, there were no attacks from the enemy and likewise with the American forces. As a matter of fact, I am even happy when it rains.

Some of the crazy things I've done! When I was about 12 years of age, I spent a vacation of two weeks with my uncle in Greensville, New Jersey. Years later and when out of the Army when very depressed, I went to Greensville and looked for the place that I had vacationed in. I was so depressed that psychologically I looked for the place where I had known some moments of happiness. I consider this a crazy thing to do because of the great distance I traveled to find nothing there. I found the area, but I didn't find the house.

N–4. What did you learn from this experience? [*Encouraging evaluation and formulation of meaning. The nurse should follow through, if possible, and try together to understand its significance.*]

P–5. I learned that my reasoning was wrong—reminiscing is good to think about happy moments. I stabbed a cat about 10 or 12 times to impress my friends, the Junior Rams. My youth as a whole was an unhappy one. Another crazy thing I used to do was to dye my hair different colors. And I used to give everything away: papers, money. I just couldn't control myself. [*He seems to want to know what the nurse thinks about him and how "awful" he is.*]

N–6. When was this? [*Placing event in time.*]

P–7. After I got out of the Army, I went through my savings of $4000. It took me about a year and a half to do this. I make every effort I can at restoring my morale. Every night here at the hospital I play pinochle, although I can only last one game—then I get nervous and tense. That's my limit.

In basic training in the Army I had to carry the rifle on my shoulder. A pain in the shoulder developed and affected the entire arm. Since I returned home from the Army and on three different occasions in cold weather, I lost complete power and movement of the right arm. [*Worth exploring concurrent interpersonal events at these times.*] I do a lot of talking to myself out loud.

N–8. What do you talk about? [*Exploring. Encouraging description.*]

P–9. Oh, about everything; seems I have to do a lot of rehearsing—before I come out with things—I need to be careful of myself. [*Worth exploring. If he did not rehearse, what might come out?*]

When I worked for the National City Bank as an IBM operator, I had to quit the job because of the pressure the job developed.

N–10. Could you describe this? [*Encouraging description.*]

P–11. I got headaches; the machines were noisy, but I worried about doing accurate work. I got the job myself. I worked there only a couple of weeks. Another job I lost as a result—the employer said was nervousness—he, the employer, fired me—it was a church job. I have become exasperated from losing jobs and friends as a result of my illness.

Another way that I try to increase my morale is by taking special enjoyment in eating breakfasts. The reason for that is because breakfasts consist of cereal and milk. I like this, but the other food I don't care for. I like the extra nourishment; my weight has increased to 165 pounds.

We bring some bread, crackers, and so forth, up on the porch, and I take enjoyment from giving it to the birds. They always eat every bit and never leave a mess on the porch.

Now our time is up—remember you promised, and I'm getting nervous.

N–12. Okay. [*Accepting.*]

(Nurse and patient walked to the door, and he said he was going to try to work on something in the occupational therapy shop for his mother for Mother's Day.)

Perhaps it would be worth exploring his "nervousness" with the nurse. It may be resulting from his concern about what he feels are her feelings about him. He seems to anticipate her disapproval. When he does not get it, he seems to get anxious. She might want to explore with him whether this might be so.

She might also want to respond sometimes with "What's so crazy (or bad or wrong) about that?" (as when he went back to New Jersey—it was inconvenient perhaps, but not "crazy"). What is worth noting is not that the things he has done are "crazy" or "wrong" but that he has to go to *extremes*: (1) stabbing a cat to impress his friends and (2) going all the way back to an event that occurred when he was 12 to recall a few moments of happiness.

Eighteenth Hour

P–1. What time is it?

N–2. Twenty minutes of one. [*Giving information.*]

P–3. We're doing okay here. We had a party last night, and the night before I stacked up about 16 packages of cigarettes.

N–4. How are you feeling? [*Encouraging description and evaluation. Better worded, "What are your feelings?"*]

P–5. I'm kind of worried about not getting a visitor this afternoon—I guess I can't take being let down. Other people have things to do regarding my mental illness. Like Jane S.—I can't take it. My brain seems to get tired quickly and can't be burdened.

N–6. So I can understand what you mean, would you explain more fully? [*Exploring. "Explain" and "mean" tend to be intimidating. "Understand" could be replaced by "follow." "Would you describe this more fully so that I can follow?"*]

P–7. I can't concentrate on two things at once or can't talk with anyone too long. That's why I wanted to cut our time to half-hour periods.

At the meal table I left the table where they talk so much. I left, but today I went back again. They discuss the hospital—normal conversation. Sometimes I think, but now I have to stop thinking. In a movie I used to concentrate on the movie—now I can't do that.

N–8. How long did you stay in the movie last night? [*Exploring.*]

P–9. About 15 minutes; it was the kind of picture I like, but I couldn't concentrate in the movie for more than 15 minutes. If I force myself to concentrate on something too long, I get a headache. Sometimes I feel like giving up, and sometimes I wish I was dead. Today, so far today, I feel pretty good. They bring parties in here, and I actually resent them.

N–10. Why? [*Requesting an explanation. Better worded, "What happens to bring about this feeling?"*]

P–11. It's a break away from routine and it upsets my equilibrum—so I resent the parties. [*This seems reasonable—he can cope with the expected but not the unexpected.*] I made two pot holders for Mother's Day for my mother in the O.T. shop this morning.

(He got them out of his pocket and handed them to the nurse.)

N–12. They are very nice. The color is bright [red], and they will be useful. [*Giving approval. Making an observation. The first part could be omitted.*]

P–13. It made me sick to make them—had a headache—wanted to be alone, and sometimes I get so upset I can't even think. I'm afraid of losing my ability to think right or correct and fearful that I may lose control over myself.

N–14. Do you want to tell me more about this? [*Exploring. Encouraging description. Most appropriate.*]

P–15. Yes; I do things that I shouldn't do—such as the time I went to New Jersey. That was a matter of losing control. I shouldn't do a thing like that—that vacation I had in New Jersey really wasn't anything.

N–16. You're beginning to evaluate experiences realistically. [*The nurse seems to be indirectly agreeing and offering approval, whereas further exploration would be more appropriate. Was this event as "crazy" or "wrong" as he thinks?*]

P–17. Yes, I'm very happy to be in the hospital where I'm understood and out of the way of my friends. I still can't let anyone touch my shoulders, as they are extremely sensitive. The shoulder and arms jump when someone touches them, and I get extremely nervous. I often feel that I don't want to bother anybody. I want to be alone and sometimes become annoyed with people.

N–18. What are the things that annoy you? [*Encouraging description.*]

P–19. Light cigarettes, ask for a cigarette. My steadiness is very easily shaken. It's like what I explained. The routine I can get used to, and I can settle myself, but when something happens out of the routine, I get easily shaken up. Any kind of pressure seems to make me angry. [*Worth exploring. The nurse might say, "Being bothered by others causes you to* *feel nervous and pressured; then you become angry. Let's explore this further."*]

This week it isn't so bad. Last Sunday I expected visitors, and they didn't come. Today the same thing. I get built up for it, and if they don't come, I'll be thrown off. [*His feelings about disappointment are worth exploring further. Perhaps he could express the anger he feels.*]

Routine days help to keep me calm. I was playing cards yesterday, and I lasted one game—then I have to quit. I like all the greenery here in ____. My family and I lived in two houses that had plant-filled yards, and I loved to walk through them. Whenever pressure is on me, I feel violent and get (violent) headaches—tense. [*The nurse should follow this up. It seems to tie in with feelings toward the father that he cannot acknowledge, e.g., "Pressure makes you angry."*]

In the Army I became used to a lot of greenery, and I missed it terribly when I came home. When the pressure is on, I feel weak and miserable.

N–20. What causes the pressure? [*Encouraging description.*]

P–21. Maintaining a lengthy conversation or being forced to think or when I force myself to think or reading a book. I can't even read a paragraph—it's too much of a strain.

N–22. Do you read the newspaper? [*Bringing up a rather unimportant detail. What needs recognition is his anxiety—only lessening his anxiety will be of help. Forcing himself to try to concentrate will only aggravate his problems.*]

P–23. Yes, I read Walter Winchell in the *Mirror,* Suzie's column, and the short stories in the paper. What time is it?

N–24. It's 1:20. Now, let's see what we talked about today. [*Giving information. Reviewing.*]

(During the review when nurse got to visitors' not coming, he elaborated.)

P–25. When I talked with my mother last night, I told her not to promise to come unless she could really make it, as I get all keyed up for the visit and if she disappoints me, I get depressed. I can't take it.

N–26. Did she say she'd come today? [*Seeking clarification.*]

P–27. Yes.

N–28. Last Sunday when they couldn't make it, you seemed to handle it quite well. [*Giving approval. Actually he may have had many unexpressed feelings about last Sunday. To give her approval would only indicate to him her lack of perception of his feelings.*]

P–29. Yeah.

(He walked to the door.)

N–30. I'll see you Friday. [*Giving information.*]

P–31. Thanks—thanks very much.

It would seem that Mr. G. is severely anxious. Peplau[1] describes anxiety by the following diagrams (the circle represents one's normal range of awareness):

Slight anxiety increases one's perceptual field. One is more alert and perceptive than usual.

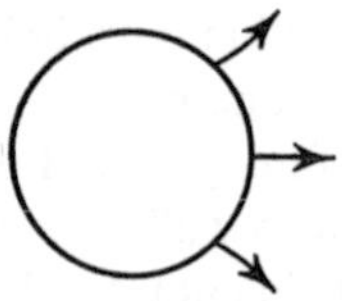

Moderate anxiety decreases awareness, e.g., the person may not hear when someone speaks to him.

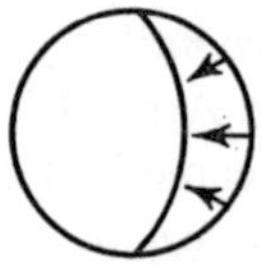

Severe anxiety causes the individual to be even less aware. He focuses on a few minute details and is unable to think about other things.

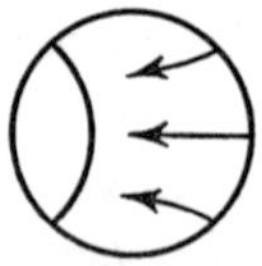

In panic, the details are blown up all out of proportion to reality. The patient loses control.

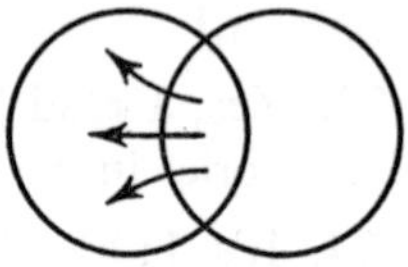

Nineteenth Hour

P–1. I haven't been feeling very well.

N–2. Could you tell me about this? [*Exploring. Encouraging description.*]

P–3. I have it written down. When I write things down, I try to make my statements as complete as possible.

Very often I feel mentally like I am some place else or like I'm on a

[1] Adapted from material presented at a workshop, "Orientation to Modern Psychiatric Nursing," by Hildegard E. Peplau (Rutgers–the State University of New Jersey) at the New Jersey State Hospital, Greystone Park, April 2–13, 1956.

cloud. The interviewing sessions that we have, if they are over half an hour, they tend to ruin my day. As I go on, I'll tell you why. Another job I lost was a job with Bickford's Cafeteria. I dated a girl there named A. and made her records—recordings. And a fellow named T. I imagined was putting the pressure on me. I imagined that he was thinking of me, and that is a sort of pressure. [*Worth exploring—thinking what of him?*] And so I quit the job, saying I was sick. Later on I received a get-well card. It was signed, "Love." [*This seems to make him anxious. Looking into this would seem of value.*] I was too sick to concentrate on her. I have been temperamental since our last interviewing session. I'll go on to tell you why I'm never sure now of whether I'm saying, thinking, or doing the right thing. [*Worth exploring. "Right thing"—what things are "right" and what are "wrong"?*] I can't maintain conversation for longer than a couple of minutes. I hope you realize how much of a strain it is for me to talk to you in our sessions, especially about things I want to forget and more painful to remember.

N–4. I realize this is hard work for you. This is done with the thought of trying to help you. [*Accepting. Giving information about the purpose of the relationship.*]

P–5. Yes, I know. It's later on after the interview. I'm exhausted. The brain is exhausted. I realize when I'm feeling better that I can't sing, and when I make recordings I only make a fool of myself.

N–6. I know it must be difficult for you to say this—you are being much more realistic in your statements. [*Accepting. The nurse should not overdo this—she has never heard him sing. Besides, it is unlikely that it is the quality of his singing that causes him to feel he "made a fool of himself."*]

P–7. Yes, you handle this information as a nurse, and I can talk with you straight from the shoulder. Often after our sessions I have to take aspirins because I get a pain in the back of my head and I also feel irritated.

N–8. The things you talk about are stressful. [*Restating. Reflecting.*]

P–9. I heard my sister's voice say she needs my help, but when I talk to her over the 'phone, she tells me she doesn't need any help. I heard the voice in C.T. this morning about 11 A.M. I haven't heard any voices for about two weeks.

N–10. What does this mean to you? [*Encouraging evaluation and description of perception. "Mean" tends to be intimidating. Perhaps the nurse might ask, "What feelings does this create?"*]

P–11. I called her on the phone, and she said she doesn't need me, and once before she needed help and didn't ask for help.

N–12. When did you talk with her? [*The nurse might have* ***restated,***

"You're not sure what to believe. You think she might need help even though she says she doesn't." Placing event in time.]

P–13. I was talking with her yesterday afternoon. Oh, I didn't get visitors yesterday. The limousine service was going to another hospital instead of here, and they didn't pick them up. They made a mistake.

N–14. This hurt you. [*Verbalizing the implied. Most appropriate.*]

P–15. Yes, it hurt me very much.

(He had tears in his eyes. Another nurse stopped to talk. The nurse introduced the patient to her.) [*If the nurse had not been interrupted, she might have said, "Let's explore this more fully." It would appear that there is a connection here. Others have always seemed to expect too much from him; yet he cannot rely on their meeting any of his expectations, even reasonable ones.*]

P–16. I would like very much to walk in the grass in the pleasant sunny weather we are having, but I realize that this is an Army whim or notion and just one more of my Army idiosyncrasies that have stuck to me. I have never reverted to civilian life. Patients often try to converse with me, and I have to walk away. [*What might happen?*]

Sometimes I have to sit at another lunch table if there is too much conversation going on. I can't help listening, but it upsets me to listen. That is why I have to sit at another table. After our sessions I often catch myself talking to myself. See how it affects me?

N–17. Yes. What do you say? [*Accepting. Encouraging description. But does the nurse see?*]

P–18. I don't remember, but I'll make it a point to write it down. Every day I walk and pace the floor until I am exhausted with walking, or my legs no longer can walk.

N–19. You're tired? [*Restating. It would seem that he feels the need to tire himself to the point of exhaustion in order to find rest.*]

P–20. Yes, I'm tired out. After our sessions I take to walking faster. What time is it?

N–21. It's 1:30. [*Giving information.*]

P–22. That's it then.

N–23. Maybe someday we can go for a walk. [*Suggesting tentative action.*]

P–24. Oh, could we? I'd love that.

N–25. When the doctor gives permission. [*Qualifying. Making the limits known.*]

P–26. I wouldn't run away or anything.

N–27. Tell me, why do you think you're here? Now think about this. [*Testing.*]

N–28. To keep me from doing the crazy things I do on the outside—

that's about 50 per cent, and the other 50 per cent is to help me by isolating me from stress and strain. I'll walk you to the door. Thanks for coming.

The only problem to even consider right now is his anxiety—his fear of losing control. This needs exploration. Encouraging him to describe these feelings in detail is indicated.

Twentieth Hour

Mr. G.'s physician wrote an order giving a nursing assistant and the nurse permission to take him for a walk on the grounds and to visit the canteen. The patient was waiting when the nurse arrived and said, "I was hoping you wouldn't disappoint me." They walked around the grounds, and he asked various questions and admired the flowers and asked about various buildings he saw in the distance. When they arrived at the canteen, he asked the nurse to sit down. He proceeded through the cafeteria line and came back with coffee. He paid the cashier with canteen coupons and had no apparent difficulty in making decisions. He sat down, lit a cigarette, smiled, and said, "Gee, this is great." Mr. G. excused himself and purchased a carton of cigarettes and a Mother's Day card. He had three cups of coffee, and the last time he went through the cafeteria line he purchased coffee and sandwiches to take to the ward for some of his friends. When they returned to the ward, he talked about some of the "crazy" things he did before coming to the hospital and what he should do on discharge—become a taxi driver, for instance. He appeared a bit tense. When they returned, he thanked the nurse profusely and said, "You just don't know what this means to me." The nurse told him she would see him Monday and that he should write down his feelings about the trip to the canteen so it could be discussed next time. He was looking forward to a visit from his parents that week end.

Twenty-first Hour

P–1. I had visitors yesterday—I had a ball; they brought me Jello and things—my mother and sister, Georgia.

N–2. You were pleased to see them. [*Reflecting his feelings.*]

P–3. Yes, I was relieved. I haven't had visitors in months. I was pleased to see them. [*Worth exploring. Had he feared they had abandoned him?*]

N–4. How do you feel now? [*Encouraging evaluation and description. Ask, "What are your feelings now?"*]

P–5. I'm steadier. When I was sick, I gave into impulses.

N–6. When you were sick? [*Restating. He may think she is testing him.*]

P–7. When I was sicker than I am now—now I don't give way to impulses. When we went to the canteen, I had an impulse to run away, but I didn't.

N–8. When did you feel this impulse—when we were out? [*Placing event in time. Perhaps the nurse could just say, "Tell me about this."*]

P–9. When you pointed out the high school. I'm stronger now, and I'm positive that I wouldn't run away. That's why I prefer seeing my visitors in the dining room, because when I was out with the visitors, I felt like running away. That's because my relatives don't take any chances—they see me inside. [*He has difficulty distinguishing his own motives from those of others.*] I miss my own neighborhood—most of the day I'm bored—I can't get comfortable and sleep in the chairs like other patients do. I don't like the meals here. I'm only used to my mother's special way of cooking. The meals are only something to break the monotony. The bathroom stinks because there is no deodorant, and every time I go in there, I feel like vomiting. Oh yes, when you took me to the canteen Friday, I was excited, and there was a slight loss of control of my hands.

N–10. Explain this more fully so that I can understand. [*Exploring. Encouraging description. "Explain" tends to be intimidating. "Tell me more about this so that I can follow."*]

P–11. When I was in the Army, I subconsciously began to train my hands—so they would work quicker than the eye. So that's when my hands began to work on their own initiative. So, what developed—whenever I want to suppress the other person, my hands go automatically for the throat. [*Quite revealing. No wonder he is anxious.*] That's what happened when I went after my sister. When I saw the high school, I felt a little nervous. When I lose control of my hands, I feel violent—like I would attack someone without provocation.

N–12. You are aware that you have to learn to control this feeling? [*Advising. Moralizing. Only as he explores the feeling and grasps its signficance will fear of this behavior change. "Control" is not the answer.*]

P–13. Yes—I learned this in the Army, and the habits I learned—I have to wake up my brain and change these habits.

N–14. Relearn. [*Restating.*]

P–15. Yes. When my visitors went home yesterday, my brain started racing again or thinking fast.

N–16. Thinking—what about? [*Exploring.*]

P–17. Thinking about what I had said to my mother and sister. I was repeating my words—talking to myself—to see if I said things with the proper emphasis. [*Worth exploring.*]

N–18. After thinking about this—[*Giving general lead. But she is jumping ahead too fast. She might have asked, "Proper emphasis?"*]

P–19. But I repeat words—it gets a grip on me—like a record that plays over and over again. I'm under a sort of control—obsessed with previous conversation.

N–20. What were you obsessed with in your visit yesterday? [*Encouraging description.*]

P–21. Mostly about my niece. My sister wants to enroll her in the Holy Name School. My sister asked me what to do. She had to make the decision by today—Monday. I told her it's too late to enroll her. [*Is he concerned that his advice might not be taken, i.e., not considered worthwhile?*] They brought me things including potato salad from the delicatessen. I had a strange feeling of going off the ward to the O.T. and C.T. shop.

N–22. What was this strange feeling like? [*Encouraging description.*]

P–23. Fearful, afraid—just the idea of going off the ward.

N–24. What do you attribute this feeling to? [*Encouraging description. Seeking source.*]

P–25. Mostly familiar—I'm familiar here on the ward—unwilling to leave. There I feel strange, that I'm losing my grip. I feel wound up because when I went to the canteen I sensed that I was beginning to unwind.

N–26. I don't understand what you mean? [*Seeking clarification. Better worded, "I don't follow what you're saying."*]

P–27. I was comfortable at the canteen. At times, I'm comfortable here. [*Worth exploring. What kind of things make him less than comfortable? What "unfamiliar" things happen? Apparently he needs to know what is expected of him.*]

I had a nightmare on Friday night. An unidentified man was chasing me with a pickax, and I woke up screaming. Saturday night I had some sort of a nightmare, but I forgot that one. When I was sick, I bought three expensive suits and threw them away without even wearing them once.

N–28. What did this mean to you? [*Encouraging evaluation. Perhaps she could say, "Tell me more about this."*]

P–29. I bought them because they attracted me. It's strange, but I threw them away—I got an impulse that I was bored with them, lost their attraction, and I threw them away.

Lately it's been more difficult for me to smile—stiff face—the last couple of weeks I feel a little stiff-faced. [*The nurse might explore this. Is it more than tension? What might he be afraid to express?*]

I'll eventually become the master of these impulses and control them. My brain seems to get tired easily, and when it does, my whole body gets tired. I have a suggestion—the best day to go to the canteen would be Wednesday.

N–30. I'll be away Wednesday. I won't have time to go out until Friday, and this will depend entirely on whether we get permission from the doctor. [*Giving information, noting conditions and necessary limitations.*]

P–31. Okay.

N–32. As long as you have these impulses, we'll have to take a nursing assistant with us, and this is to help you. Do you understand? [*Giving further information about limits.*]

P–33. Yes, you want to help me until I master this impulse feeling about not running away. Oh yes, I walked out on Mr. W.'s remotivation group that meets on Thursday afternoon—after only 10 minutes went by. I couldn't take the mental strain, and I was forced to think too deep.

N–34. What were they discussing? [*Encouraging description.*]

P–35. Hotels.

N–36. Did it remind you of something? [*Exploring. A good try.*]

P–37. No, because I've had no business with hotels. I almost started a fight on Friday. [*Worth exploring further. Does it bother him to be called on?*]

N–38. Tell me about it. [*Encouraging description. Most appropriate response.*]

P–39. A fellow was talking to the O.T. therapist, and this fellow was talking with her, and I went over and told him to come on, and he said he wasn't holding up anything—the thing for me to do was to mind my own business—I almost lost control. [*Worth exploring. What did he fear he might do? What were his feelings toward the other patient in this situation?*]

When I came back from the canteen, I felt shaken up in a happy way—I was shaken up, but I was happy.

P–40. I have a blank expression, and it's hard for people to understand. When I went to the canteen, I felt good—I was free to master my impulses. [*He seems to feel that others believed he would not "act out" these impulses.*]

N–41. We're trying to help you. I want to know about these impulses—when you get them and how you feel. Will you write them down so we can discuss them? [*Encouraging description. Appropriate.*]

P–42. Yes, yes, I will.

N–43. If you have these impulses toward me, I want you to tell me so that we can talk about them. Will you do this? [*Encouraging description.*]

P–44. Yes. I know you want to help me master them. [*The nurse* *should put emphasis on knowing more about them, rather than mastery of them.*]

N–45. I'll see you Friday, and after we work, provided the doctor gives permission, we'll go to the canteen for a cup of coffee, and we'll take an aide with us. [*Giving information. Tentatively suggesting possible action.*]

P–46. Fine. Thanks, thanks very much.

The nurse seems to be on the right track. Now he is finally getting down to the real sources of his anxiety—the fear of acting out his hostility. It will take time, but he needs to learn that feelings are not equal to deeds, that feelings are not right or wrong, that it is all right to feel angry toward other people. The nurse should not push this idea, however. He has a long way to go first. She can help by getting him to describe in detail for now. Later she can point out similarities between the various situations in which these impulses are aroused. Better still, perhaps he will be able to see the similarities between these situations himself. But first she must collect a series of these events in detail—times when he has felt the impulse to strangle, for instance. She will want to know what led up to the incident, who was involved, exactly what was said by the participants, his feelings during the event, the outcome, and his feelings following the experience.

Twenty-second Hour

P–1. In my notes, I tried to fully explain each statement. [*Silence is the interpersonal technique during this sequence.*] When my brain thinks fast and I can't stop it, I get dizzy. I feel depressed and unhappy, and I don't quite know why. When we eat in the mess hall for 50 minutes, it depresses me to be there so long—you see I'm trying to search for things that depress me to tell you—I find it difficult to sit in a position for more than one minute. I'm depressed because it's taking my sister a long time to get married. I still walk and pace the floor most of the day. I'm subscribed to a newspaper, but when I get it, I only read a couple of paragraphs, and then I give it away.

My mother gave me a roll of nickles ($2 worth) and four quarters. I got an impulse and gave the four quarters away. [*This impulse is worth exploring in detail.*] I am depressed because of a constant pain in my side around the vicinity of the stomach.

I am depressed because coffee is a most important part of my meal and the coffee they serve here is too inexpensive. I believe the coffee is to blame for this pain in my side.

I am sneezing now more than any other period in my life. I am depressed with living with this particular group of men. They sneeze and cough and blow their noses in the dining room while eating. I still can't play more than one game of cards. I still have not the patience to do anything in the O.T. in the way of a project. I still walk constantly as a resistance to my problems. I'm still depressed and worried about my sister Mary. I still think about my war experiences. [*Perhaps this would have been an appropriate time to summarize briefly and then encourage description, e.g., "You've been telling me the things that depress you. Which would you say are the most important?" Then, "Perhaps you and I should look more closely at those you've selected. It's only as these situations are fully explored that their significance will become clear. Tell me about each of them in greater detail."*] I still think in terms of suicide.

N–2. What do you think about suicide? [*Encouraging description.*]

P–3. Where to get poison and how to do the job, so I need to get poison.

N–4. You don't want to live? [*Verbalizing the implied for verification.*]

P–5. When I'm sick, I don't want to live. If I get sick again, I want to be prepared. When I was sick, I searched in vain for poison. I paid $15 a bottle for poison, and I took it. I waited to see what would happen, and it didn't affect me. It turned out to be some photograph fluid.

N–6. You feel this way now? [*Encouraging evaluation. "This way" is vague. Better worded, "What are your present feelings?"*]

P–7. Sometimes I do, and sometimes I don't. My mind seems to be made up to one thing—I need to have the poison just in case. I don't feel like committing suicide now. When I was sick the last time, I needed something, and I couldn't get it.

N–8. Will you tell me when you feel this way? [*Encouraging description of perceptions at time of occurrence. Appropriate. She might also suggest exploring "the last time" he "felt like" taking poison. E.g., what events led to this decision? Where was he and with whom? What were his thoughts and feelings? What did he do and what were his feelings when he was unsuccessful?*]

P–9. Yes. I still feel more like I'm in Korea than a civilian. I had a nightmare Monday night. I only remember that a man was chasing me—that's all I remember. He was quite a distance away, and I couldn't distinguish the features. I started running; then I woke up.

I'm still tired in the mornings and I think I could do with a couple of more hours of sleep. I feel a little cranky in the morning after getting out of bed. The O.T. and C.T. I don't enjoy, and the time seems to go by slowly. I still can't put things out of my mind.

N–10. What sort of things out of your mind? [*Exploring. Encouraging description.*]

P–11. Most often it's a song.

N–12. What does the song remind you of? [*Going beyond the data. He has not suggested that it reminds him of anything. It would have been better to ask "A particular song?" or "Tell me more."*]

P–13. It might mean something special to me—"You Don't Know Me" —it seemed to be expressing my own sentiments.

N–14. Do you feel that you know about yourself? [*Testing. The nurse could ask, "In what way?"*]

P–15. No, I don't, and I promised myself that I will take time to make decisions, and that's why I'm glad I'm in the hospital. I have time to think things out.

We had a party Monday night, and I don't enjoy them. They seem to upset me because they are not part of the routine. I think having the party caused the nightmare. Also I think maybe our interview. Monday afternoon may have had something to do with my having a nightmare. [*The nurse might want to explore the possibility that something in particular from Monday's discussion caused him concern. She might ask, "What were your thoughts after Monday's conversation?"*] It seems that when my brain is strained or weakened that anything can happen. The afternoons are the slowest-going part of my day. I'm uncomfortable because I can't sleep or sit in the chairs like the rest of the men do. In the O.T., I started to make a rug but couldn't finish it. I made two pot holders for my mother for Mother's Day, but they were stolen before I could give them to her. I ate my fill at the party. I am eating very well. Recently I got an impulse not to take the medication. I drank the water and kept the medication in my hand. Mr. K. [R.N.] caught me and put me on liquid medication. I had to talk with the doctor to get back on pill medication again. I will never do that again because I can't stand liquid medication.

When the canteen came to the ward, I bought a guy two bags of peanuts when I needed the money for myself—you see, I lost control again. [*His "lost control" is worthy of exploration. Is he saying that giving is undesirable—even abnormal—especially when it is unlikely to bring any return? Perhaps he feels so empty, with so many unmet needs of his own, that to give is to deprive himself even further.*]

I can play one game of pool before reactions—then, of course, I stop playing. I am uncomfortable because my mouth is dry and sour-tasting because of the pill medication. An aide told me when I first came here that I was sloppy, but now I've improved. Sometimes writing these notes makes me dizzy. [*Twice today he has mentioned dizziness. The nurse can help him to see this as an indication of anxiety and encourage him to describe situations in which it occurs and to explore in what way these situations are similar.*]

My system for eating is to eat a big breakfast and a small dinner and supper—to do it any other way would depress me. Since I got that carton of cigarettes, when I last went to the canteen with you, I got impulses and gave away six packs. [*Again he speaks of getting "impulses." The three separate situations could be explored together, along with the accompanying thoughts and feelings.*]

My sister asked me a question when she visited me—the question was that she thought the parochial school in our area was taking only children whose parents contributed to the church. She has a child named Linda who will be old enough to be sent to school this year. When she visited me, I gave her an incomplete answer. After they had gone, and I promised to call my mother on the telephone the following Thursday, and so the following Monday I got a terrific impulse to telephone, and I did. I told my sister the best thing to do was to go to church and say "Hello" to the priest on the way out and also to contribute. My action of calling beforehand did not seem normal to me. It would have been normal to my personal judgment to wait until Thursday as I promised to call on Thursday.

N–16. You wanted to get this off your mind? [*Offering tentative explanation. The nurse might have verbalized the implied, "Are you suggesting that it was abnormal not to wait?" And if the answer was affirmative, ask, "I don't quite follow. In what way is this so unusual?"*]

P–17. It would have been normal to wait. When I walk with my hands alerted—they are always unclasped and ready for action—this is not normal—the hands are ready to spring. I keep expressing myself with my hands, and this is not the normal way I express myself. It is a sign of a dangerous personality. Sometimes my hands pop up into the air from my side for no reason. I'm in best form with everything happening on a daily schedule. I get upset with any happenings that are days apart. I don't think I mentioned that when I choked my sister to the point that she blacked out—that I felt an abnormal pleasure of killing. [*This event should be explored in detail when it comes up again.*]

N–18. Will you tell me when you feel this way? [*Encouraging description of perceptions at time of occurrence.*]

P–19. Yes, yes, I will. Last time when we talked I got upset—maybe you noticed—I felt my hands going for your throat.

N–20. You did? [*Seeking confirmation of what he just said.*]

P–21. Yes, but you don't have to worry, I have control of myself. I wouldn't hurt you.

N–22. When you feel this way, you should talk about it then. [*Giving advice. Rather than "you should," the nurse could say "I'd like you to. . . ."*]

P–23. Yes. Is it time to go?

N–24. Yes. [*By not summarizing, the nurse allows the patient to con-*

tinue bringing up anxiety-provoking material for which no time is left to explore or to resolve in any way.]

(The patient had permission from the doctor to go to the canteen for coffee. An aide went along. It was a pleasant trip with general conversation.)

Twenty-third Hour

P–1. I made a 'phone call to my home. Every time I do I feel dizzy and my mind seems to be spinning and—I got into a couple of arguments on the ward.

N–2. You get upset when you call home? [*Reflecting.*]

P–3. I suddenly think too fast for my brain, and it upsets me.

N–4. I can't follow what upsets you when you call home. [*Seeking clarification.*]

P–5. I'm upset with the way my sister Mary was treated. She didn't get enough help in her life. When a person accuses another person of doing foul things—I imagined my father was trying to murder me—it's like a wall between me and my family. My sickness has lost me the friendship of my father and brother-in-law. I don't think they are going to forgive me for the things I've said.

N–6. You are expressing feelings. It is important for you to express these feelings. [*Making an observation. But it is impressions he is describing. What happened to give him these impressions?*]

P–7. Sometimes I get the feeling that I shouldn't call up. I have a feeling that I should help them.

N–8. You've identified a problem. [*Making an observation. Has he? If so, it needs to be clearly defined. Again, the nurse needs to explore what happened to give him the impression that he should not call or that his family needs help.*]

P–9. Yes, but I want to talk about my trip to the canteen last Friday. When we got back to the ward, I seemed to be going to pieces. I believe the sweat was part of the strain. We stepped out into a different environment. I didn't want to talk because it was too much of a strain, and on the way back my hands were stiff. I almost couldn't talk and couldn't realize my answers or couldn't think up my answers. My face was stiff like the skin is hard—and, I sensed that I couldn't smile. When I got back to the ward, I found myself talking to myself. I was repeating sentences I had said during our outing and wondering if the things I said received the correct understanding. When I got back to the ward, I had a sort of headache. [*"Correct understanding" might be explored. Is it that he expects to be misunderstood?*]

N–10. This caused tension. [*Verbalizing the implied.*]

P–11. Yes. When I got back to the ward, I began pacing—fast, in an effort to walk off my mental strain. I had a feeling of fitness to kill—my mind just seemed to black out—my will was weak when I gave away a sheet of the newspaper I had bought. I got an impulse to give him the newspaper and it got the best of me. [*"A feeling of fitness to kill" should be explored more fully. Did it follow the "impulse" to give away the paper?*]

N–12. What do you feel that you should have said when the man asked you for the paper? [*Reflecting.*]

P–13. I should have said I'll save it for him.

N–14. You have difficulty saying "no"? [*Verbalizing the implied.*]

P–15. I want to be liked and accepted, and I'm willing to give to be accepted. I do this to keep a friend. I'm afraid of losing one.

N–16. If you have to go too far to keep a friend, is it worth it? [*Encouraging evaluation. However, the question is worded so that it almost insists on a negative reply. Perhaps the nurse should try to discover the meaning to the patient of the word "friend" and the source of his impression that they are easily lost.*]

P–17. That's what I say, it wasn't worth it.

Now I want to tell you about when I wanted to kill myself. When we got back to the building and you asked me to talk with Mr. K. [R.N.], I wanted to kill myself and wished I was dead because I couldn't smile. [*"Couldn't smile" is worth exploring. What led up to the feeling? What is it that he anticipates with dread in unfamiliar environments?*] I was so upset. I'm requesting that whenever we go to the canteen that you bring me directly to the ward—even though I'm enjoying going to the canteen, but it's a strain on me. I was so anxious to get back on the ward. This is a new environment I've got to get used to slowly.

I'm depressed because my ears hurt me, and I seem to be dragging my right leg. My partial rupture is on the right side, and my right arm hangs heavier—sometimes my shoulder pains. My ear trouble may have something to do with the fact that I strain my ears whenever I force myself on the toilet. I'm constipated most of the time. And I can twitch or move my ears as I sometimes do when it amuses others. I still jump whenever anyone touches my right shoulder. When I can get a container of coffee on the ward, the men nearly always ask for and get three-fourths of it. I get annoyed at myself for giving it away. [*His feelings about "giving away" might be further explored. One gets the feeling that it is as though he loses part of himself each time.*]

I lose contact with reality when I watch motion pictures—on Tuesday and Thursday nights. When they do show movies, it weakens me, and I suffer twice a week and I suffer. We're locked in and I have to watch the movie. [*The nurse might explore what he is referring to as "loss of contact with reality." What takes place?*]

I'm depressed because my feelings are still hurt by Jane S. I feel a little better because I wrote a letter to each member of my immediate family—on May 16th and 17th. This May 19th I got up out of bed feeling grouchy. I sense or feel about myself a greater incentive to make notes because of our going to the canteen. I've noticed that I've been asking for aspirins an average of two every two days for headaches. I noticed I get the headaches after a mental strain. [*The nurse could ask for examples of what he calls "mental strain."*]

I used to imagine that my father was trying to kill me. I remember that there were three occasions on which I thought he was trying to kill me. Of the three, I can remember only one. It was when I was working with him with a brick company that he is still working for.

N–18. What happened? [*Encouraging description of perceptions.*]

P–19. He asked me to back up a truck on the top floor of a pier. I backed the truck up successfully, but I later learned that the truck had faulty brakes. [*The incident described lacks detail. What led him to believe that this was intentional, for example?*] I used to imagine my mother was overly fond of me and didn't want me to get married and that she seen to it that I was too busy with business to have time for girls and that is a fact that I was always too busy with business to bother with girls. [*Is he saying that there is a connection between the father's "intent" and the mother's "overfondness" for him?*]

I woke up Saturday with my infected eye closed. It was 15 minutes before I could get it open. I'm putting compresses on it.

(Nurse and patient talked about going to the canteen that week and agreed that the next day would be a good time since it was usually crowded on Wednesday. The patient asked if the aide had to go with them and was told it was the physician's order.)

If the patient is not too anxious to focus, the nurse should encourage description in detail of the major interpersonal difficulties he brings up in each hour, especially family relationships. This is one of few times he has mentioned his mother and his relationship with her.

Twenty-fourth Hour

P–1. You know the last time when we went out to the canteen—when we got back, I was sweating—not because of the heat but because of the pressure.

N–2. Pressure. Tell me about this feeling in detail, so I can follow what you mean. [*Focusing. Encouraging description of perceptions. ". . . follow what you're saying."*]

P–3. Yes, well, it worked up slowly, but I gradually couldn't help but shy away from you because for a few minutes I couldn't think.

N–4. Tell me more about the pressure buildup. [*Exploring.*]

P–5. Well, on the way back I explained how Dr. X. analyzed me correctly when he made the statement that the other ward was too fast for me. As time went by, the canteen became too fast an environment for me. I couldn't think for a time.

N–6. What incidents contributed to this feeling—led up? [*Placing events in sequence.*]

P–7. It was nice of you to ask me to go for a newspaper. When you asked me if I wanted a newspaper—I hadn't planned to get one—so this shook me up. It upsets me to be watched by an aide. It seems like I am being watched very closely, and it makes me nervous. You don't make me feel this way. You have a successful and capable approach to me.

N–8. Tension results when the aide is with us. [*Restating.*]

P–9. Yes, I definitely would not run away. I have no wish at the moment to go back to my former way of life with business people and social living. It's as if we were handcuffed together.

N–10. You and the aide? [*Seeking consensual validation.*]

P–11. Yes, it's different to be with a group, rather than with one aide and you, and, to top it off, being with the people in the atmosphere and environment of the canteen—it's something that I sense. . . .

N–12. Go on. [*Offering general lead.*]

P–13. I sense better brains working, and I feel belittled.

N–14. Belittled. [*Restating.*]

P–15. It's just that I don't think fast, and I'm among people who think fast, so I sense faster minds at work. Whenever I go to the canteen, you cannot help being interested in being involved with other people, and when I start analyzing and understanding them, this creates tension.

N–16. Several people joined us at the table, and when I introduced you to them, this made you feel nervous? [*Restating to make certain that she has grasped the idea he is attempting to convey.*]

P–17. Yes, I felt I was exposed to a healthy person and that I might say something that looks foolish—it affected me for the rest of the day. We gain by going to the canteen without getting involved with too many other individuals.

N–18. Let's summarize this experience. You felt tense because the canteen was too fast an environment. You couldn't think for a time because other individuals got into our conversation. It took too much out of you to make general conversation. Too, the aide with us made you feel that you were being watched—handcuffed to him. You've indicated that you would not run away. [*Summarizing. Most appropriate.*]

P–19. Yes, now we know that it is 50 per cent the aide and 50 per cent the environment of the canteen. So now we know what causes our trouble over there. I'm a little tense now—I have a little headache. The upper-right-hand corner of my head hurts, but my hands are O.K. [*Worthy of further exploration. Usually, when tense, he fears losing control of his hands.*]

I used to get furnished rooms, and I would get one for a day and pay a week's rent. I did this at several places for the same time. I was hopping around like a jackrabbit—now this isn't normal.

N–20. So that I can follow your thinking on this, would you tell me about the things that preceded this going about? [*Encouraging description. Placing events in sequence.*]

P–21. My father was kind of unpredictable in many ways. I couldn't think in partnership, so just talking with him gave me a headache.

N–22. And you went out? [*Verbalized the implied.*]

P–23. Yes, I couldn't seem to think. My father said I was holding a grudge. My mind was always a blank, and so I decided to live alone. I wasn't happy with the personality of my father. My father wanted to do things in an unorthodox manner. [*"Unorthodox manner" is worth exploring.*]

The last business was the vending business in apartments. He, at times, wouldn't do the collecting and would go out to the racetrack and with money from the business—we had a small business, 25 machines—but he was undependable, and unreliability is a strain on me. I'd have to do his work at times. See, I depended upon him for his electrical ability. He wouldn't repair the machines when they broke down. He'd be going out to the racetrack.

N–24. Did you talk this over with him? [*Exploring.*]

P–25. I'm not the arguing kind. I just walk out. [*Perhaps the nurse could restate, "When you are angry with your father, you feel tense, get a headache, and find it necessary to walk out."*] At the brick company I worked there before I imagined one of the employees wanted to kill me, so I wrote the boss, a millionaire, a poison-pen letter, and it cost me my job.

N–26. You imagined one of the employees was trying to kill you? [*Restating.*]

P–27. Yes, when I was in a truck and backed it up on the pier, my father was there and the boss of the brick company.

N–28. You thought they were trying to kill you? [*Reflecting.*]

P–29. I thought so. Now I'm not so sure. I would say I wasn't sick at that time—17. I don't remember feeling ill at that time, but it may have been that I was ill—at that time.

N–30. You wrote the pen letter on this one incident? [*Seeking clarification. Perhaps the nurse could have said, "Let's go over this in more detail from the beginning. It may be possible to distinguish what was real from what wasn't."*]

P–31. It's the only incident that I can remember. It must be that I was ill then and my imagination ran away with me. I have only enough mental strength to write my notes. Anything else is too much of a strain. These impulses—what makes me angry is my . . . is the way I use my hands to express myself and my lack of control over them.

N–32. Shall we talk about this? [*Giving a broad opening.*]

P–33. Well, I don't know. I'm angry because the way I lose control. Here's something that will add to our understanding. You asked me to confine my topics to my feelings, and if we run out of things to say, we would just sit. The trouble with that is that it is unbearable for me to just sit. I need to get up and walk. [*The nurse might comment, "When you are tense, you feel the need to do something physically exerting."*] This method of discussing things I don't care for—I have to reach for understanding—merely to read my notes isn't as much of a strain.

N–34. Discussing things helps me to follow. [*Giving information about the relationship. She might also restate, "Reaching for understanding creates tension."*]

P–35. It's a strain.

N–36. Our time is up. Are you feeling up to a trip to the canteen? [*Giving information. Encouraging evaluation.*]

P–37. Could we?

N–38. Yes, for a cup of coffee, and we'll try not to get involved with too many people today. [*Accepting. Tentatively planning action.*]

(The aide who went along did not join the patient and the nurse at the table for coffee. The hospital personnel were less conspicuous. On return the patient said, "This was the best trip we had." He was less tense.)

From the discussion today, the nurse can see that the patient has difficulty expressing his hostility, especially toward his father. When angry, he becomes tense and feels it necessary to remove himself from the father's presence. Then he projects this hostility to his father and fears that the latter wants to kill him. The nurse is aware, however, that the patient would gain nothing from her telling him these things. Considerable more exploration of the father-son relationship seems indicated if the patient is to grasp its significance and come to understand the manner in which it influences his present behavior.

Twenty-fifth Hour

(The patient looked over some notes he had.)

P–1. My feelings about our canteen experience—I've been experiencing a blank mind for a few minutes. This occurred on the last trip.

N–2. Do you remember when this occurred? [*Placing event in time.*]

P–3. I don't remember the exact time. At this time I experience loss of control of my hands—not complete control though. Here is another thing that hurts my feelings. I imagine that people are taking a dislike to me or are avoiding me as a result of my stiff face or look on my face.

N–4. Tell me more about this. I don't seem to notice this. [*Exploring to encourage clarification and description.*]

P–5. It's not very noticeable. I imagine that I'm losing friends because I can't smile.

N–6. You imagine. [*Restating to emphasize that this is his impression.*]

P–7. I know I'm not losing as many friends as I imagine—to a small degree. A smile draws people. Oh! Has Miss G. told you that I have managed to do a few things in the O.T. shop?

N–8. No. Tell me about them. [*Exploring.*]

P–9. I've been typing two paragraphs a day—on the stock list of tools.

N–10. What are your feelings about this? [*Encouraging evaluation.*]

P–11. I feel good about this but I become tired, and slightly irritated.

N–12. Would you describe this feeling? [*Encouraging description of perceptions.*]

P–13. The irritation—it takes a form of tenseness of the brain and a sort of twisted look on my face.

N–14. Twisted look? [*Restating to encourage clarification.*]

P–15. My face muscles tighten up. When I'm tense, I feel as though my eyes are still searching for the enemy as they did in Korea. This is difficult to understand because you wouldn't be familiar as to the way your eyes look for things in Korea. When you see a few men get killed, your eyes are on a constant watch trying to pierce the darkness—the eyes take on a special movement—coverage in all directions is important. I discovered after a month of combat that my eyes weren't blinking any more.

N–16. And you still do this? [*Verbalizing the implied for confirmation.*]

P–17. Yes, my eyes have this very special look from time to time.

N–18. I don't seem to notice anything different. [*Presenting reality.*]

P–19. And related to this, my ears are alert to hear everything. I was a very neat person before going in the Army. There I was used to heavy combat—now, an aide told me I had improved.

N–20. Your appearance. [*Verbalizing the implied.*]

P–21. I want to be neat and clean, but I can't seem to be that way. My attitude is still somewhat careless. The Army taught me to be lazy, and as a result I have a lazy approach. This will give you an idea of how I am feeling—I find it difficult to sit and wait in the mess hall for 50 minutes. This is very depressing. It takes me 10 minutes to eat, and I have to sit there 50 minutes—this is depressing. I heard a noise for about 15 minutes like a radio signal or wave.

N–22. When did you hear this? [*Placing event in time.*]

P–23. I don't remember—didn't put down the date.

N–24. Tell me more about this. [*Exploring.*]

P–25. I've heard it quite often in my life. It's like sometimes you switch on the radio and hear a sound—that's what it's like—a shrill whistle. I don't think this is imaginary.

N–26. Can you think of any incident that precedes this sound? [*Attempting to place in sequence.*]

P–27. No.

N–28. Can you associate other activity with this sound? [*Encouraging description of concurrent events.*]

P–29. No. It's like a radio signal.

N–30. What are your feelings about this? [*Encouraging evaluation and description.*]

P–31. I'm confused about this. I can't figure out what it is or what is causing this. I used to slip down in the chair to rest my back—and lay down on the floor—now I don't do this. This must have been my imagination.

N–32. Your back is feeling better? [*Verbalizing the implied.*]

P–33. Yes, there has been an improvement. I don't slip down to the floor any more.

N–34. From time to time you identify things that you thought were real and now you think they were your imagination. [*Summarizing.*]

P–35. Yes, oh yes, I'm improving. You asked me to tell you when I had feelings about wanting to die or to commit suicide. Whenever I think of the social things I have done or the friends I have lost, I feel this way.

N–36. Tell me more. [*Exploring.*]

P–37. And I feel depressed because I have lost the respect of my family. I don't have a desperate feeling about suicide; it's more of a mild feeling. The dream I had—when I eloped with Mr. K. [R.N.]—I thought the hospital authorities were looking at me and the authorities looked like a military group. When I was sick, I accused my father of trying to kill me. I accused him of increasing my insurance when he knew I was going to fight in Korea, and I called him a draft dodger.

N–38. He did this? [*Seeking clarification.*]

P–39. My mother said not.

N–40. Would you say this is imagination, as you've indicated before? [*Reflecting. Tentatively verbalizing what may be implied.*]

P–41. Yes, I think it is. It may be my imagination. I was in three fights because things I imagined bothered me.

N–42. In what way? [*Encouraging description of perceptions. Each event should be explored.*]

P–43. I imagined they had me on their minds, and I didn't like it, and I felt there would be trouble. It happened with that group of boys called the Cool Cats. I imagined so much that I hired a private detective. They weren't after me, but no one could convince me of that when I was sick. I imagined they were bothering me. I'm doing better writing about my feelings about things. This is what you want, isn't it?

N–44. Your feelings in as much detail as possible. [*Giving information about the nature and purpose of the relationship.*]

Twenty-sixth Hour

P–1. I realize that you judge the interviews by the conclusions we come to, and see what we can learn about them. Right?

N–2. Yes, to a degree. [*Accepting. Perhaps better worded, "Yes, their value lies in what you and I can learn from them."*]

P–3. So I wrote down topics we can discuss. See, I'm learning how to work with you. My imagination seems to be working again. I'm depressed because I imagined my father and brother-in-law won't drive my sister and mother out to visit me, and that is why my mother and sister come by limousine.

N–4. Tell me more as to how you feel about this. [*Exploring. Encouraging description. ". . . your feelings about this."*]

P–5. I think my father and brother-in-law have given up on me, and I think that I shouldn't go home again—I'm not making plans to go home. When I'm living at home, I seem to fail at every task I take care of. Should I go home when I get out of here?

N–6. This is a decision you must make. From what you say, you are very fond of your parents but do not like some of the things they do. [*Reflecting. Restating. Verbalizing the implied.*]

P–7. Did I tell you about how I went from one job to another?

N–8. Yes, to some extent. [*Acknowledging that this was so.*]

P–9. When I was with the family, every time I went in a business with my father I failed. I believe they are jealous of me even though they are better off than I am.

N–10. We've never discussed your feelings about your father. [*Making an observation. She could add, "Tell me about this jealousy."*]

P–11. I believe my father is capable of a nationality.

N–12. A nationality. [*Restating for the purpose of seeking clarification.*]

P–13. My father is Italian, and even though he raised me—he is distinctly Italian, and I think he is jealous because I'm Irish.

N–14. You're Irish? [*Restating. Seeking clarification.*]

P–15. You see, I changed my name. My father's name originally was C. and he changed it to J. I didn't like this, and I tried to have my name changed back to C., but I couldn't; so then I took my mother's name without the prefix. Do you understand about the meaning of the prefix? The "O" means "the descendant of"; so it was right for me to take the name of G. My mother is hurting me because she is keeping me from getting married.

N–16. Tell me about this. [*Exploring. Encouraging description.*]

P–17. A few years back she said, "I want you to be my son and I don't want you to get married." They both seem to keep me busy and find things for me to do. The business took up all my time, and the strain was too great, and they did little to relieve this. And they were always in business, and it was always like this. I was kept too busy to think about myself, and I always got sick with the heavy work load.

N–18. How do you feel toward your father as a result of this? [*Encouraging evaluation. Better worded, "What are your feelings toward . . . ?"*]

P–19. I feel as though I've been made a fool of and got nothing out of it. I got tired, general strain, and veins popped out of my legs because I stood too long.

N–20. You didn't feel that they were trying to help you? [*Encouraging evaluation, but suggesting the response. It would be worth trying, "You felt angry with him, and this made you feel tense?"*]

P–21. They had made up their minds that I was to be a bachelor. I wanted to become a married man, if only as a result of ambition. I have just about decided to go my own way. That's what my plans are at the present time. I told you that I bought a couple of rifles, and they found out about them and confiscated them—I even dared to shoot one of them.

N–22. To shoot one of them. [*Restating.*]

P–23. Both.

N–24. Is this a way to solve a problem? [*Asking for evaluation, but implying disapproval. A more appropriate response might be, "Tell me about this from the beginning. I'm not sure that I follow."*]

P–25. This is what we were taught in the service, and when I get angry, I get all tensed up and want to kill.

N–26. You're living in peacetime now. What would have happened to you if you had shot them? [*Giving information that implies disapproval. Encouraging description, but implying the threat of punishment.*]

P–27. Probably the electric chair.

N–28. How should you handle this? [*Encouraging the formulation of a plan of action. This is premature. The nurse seems to ask, "Can't you be good rather than bad?"*]

P–29. Well, I know I must rehabilitate myself to civilian living. But I was angry because my sister married a bad man, and it didn't last—only five years, then they separated.

N–30. This was her decision. [*Giving information that is meant to be reassuring. It would seem appropriate to ask, "Angry with whom?" and then explore this feeling further.*]

P–31. But she wasn't educated and didn't know what she was doing. The family is prejudiced against me because I'm part Italian. I look mostly like my father. I decided to look Italian and dyed my hair black and spent $1000 to see what it felt like to be Italian.

N–32. What did you do? [*Exploring. Encouraging description.*]

P–33. I went and lived in an Italian neighborhood and visited Italian bars.

N–34. And. . . . [*Offering a general lead.*]

P–35. I enjoyed it. My parents favored my sister Georgia and not me or Mary.

N–36. In what way? [*Encouraging description of perceptions.*]

P–37. I'm a long way behind in understanding people in relation to my age. All this happened after I got out of the service. I think I can solve all my problems with a gun. It has taken me out of reality—then I'm in another world. I'd like to tell you about two things that I did. One winter it was very icy and all over the ground. So, this O'D. was the Democratic captain in our neighborhood. He was trying to find a way to get out to the airport and, without my father's permission, I offered the use of the family car to Mr. O'D.

N–38. What was wrong about this? [*Exploring. But he has not said yet that it was wrong.*]

P–39. You see it was wrong because I also offered my father as the driver.

N–40. He could have said "no." [*Reassuring. Defending the patient.*]

P–41. But you see, after I told the man we'd take him out, I begged and begged my father to take him. And the roads were very dangerous as they were icy. My father drove the captain out to the airport, and then Mr. O'D. decided he'd take a cab back. This made my father very, very angry. This is just one more example of a loss of control of my mind, and it is another example of how I gave things away.

N–42. This appears to be a friendly gesture on your part. Your father could have said "no." [*Again seeming to defend the patient. Perhaps the nurse could sum up: "The idea seemed reasonable in the beginning, but your father saw it differently. When it ended badly, you felt you'd been taken advantage of. Is that it?"*]

P–43. But as I said, I begged him to do it. I said we can do it. So I arranged it all around. [*The "impulses" that follow seem to be quite similar to the one above. The nurse and patient could explore them together and try to see why the patient cannot say "no."*] And I impulsively gave my weights away. I only had them a month. I just lost control and gave them away, and there is no excuse for this. I worked hard and spent $80 on a gun, and I sold it for $10—so by doing this it was a crazy thing to do, and I don't know what possessed me.

We have movies here, and I'm always glad when they are over, because when I'm watching the movie, it's like losing contact with reality.

N–44. You get lost in the movie? [*Seeking consensual validation.*]

P–45. I didn't like the feeling. Our time is up.

(The nurse and the patient went to the canteen. He was self-sufficient there—went through the cafeteria line for coffee and sandwiches. Then he got a supply of cigarettes. He exchanged friendly greetings with other patients. On the way back, they talked about the feelings he was experiencing. Each time he seems to feel less tense. He told the nurse that his family disappointed him again on visiting day.)

Twenty-seventh Hour

P–1. I did the same thing as I did last week—thought you wanted more of a discussion so that we could talk about a topic and then come to some conclusions. I have several topics. I'd like to tell you how much progress I've made in the O.T. and C.T.

N–2. Go on. [*Offering a general lead.*]

P–3. In this hospital I've been doing some drawings. I started a meat board and did some typing. Now, I type for about a 15-minute period. In the C.T. I've never been interested in gymnastics, so I just pace. I'm not interested in this. The next topic: when in Korea, I learned to kill, and I sort of enjoyed it. Then when I choked my sister—when I realized it was her, I stopped.

N–4. Tell me about this. [*Exploring. Encouraging description.*]

P–5. One day she was playing the radio, TV, and phonograph all at the same time, and I asked her to play one at a time. There were some nasty remarks.

N–6. Some nasty remarks. [*Restating.*]

P–7. I don't remember the remarks. I choked her, and she almost fainted.

N–8. Almost. [*Restating. Emphasizing that she did not faint.*]

P–9. I stopped; she collapsed and almost fainted. She fell on the floor. I don't know if she ever forgave me for this.

N–10. Go on. [*Offering a general lead.*]

P–11. Georgia heard the argument, and she came down, and Mary went upstairs with her. I lost control of myself for a time.

N–12. Tell me more about losing control. [*Exploring. Encouraging description.*]

P–13. I went over to her and started choking her, and when it got to the point when I knew she needed air and I realized it was my sister, at that point, I let loose. [*Did it seem to be someone else?*]

N–14. What are your feelings about this? [*Reflecting. It would be worthwhile to explore what followed the incident: what was said or done, the manner in which his sister related to him. Such description might clarify the extent to which the event is real.*]

P–15. I feel that she hasn't forgiven me about this. She holds it against me that I gave her dog away. She found out who I gave the dog to, and she went to court to get the dog back. I think she is still angry with me for these two reasons. She has never forgiven me.

N–16. She has never forgiven you? [*Restating.*]

P–17. For one reason, she never comes to see me. Since I've been here, she hasn't visited me at all. She was frightened to death and looked very, very frightened, and she knew that she was almost killed. She looked at me unbelievingly. Sometimes I call the house, and from the telephone conversation and tone of her voice I know she is disappointed. I want to make it up to her, and I realize she loved the dog very much, and I gave the dog away.

Since I've been out of the service, I have my breaking point, and I don't have to be driven too far to want to murder someone—like my sister, when I almost choked her. The two of us were sitting in the kitchen and having coffee. At home, we hang out in the kitchen most of the time. I pushed my thumbs on her Adam's apple and pushed it all the way back to the backbone.

N–18. You thought. [*Reflecting. Emphasizing that this is his impression.*]

P–19. Yes, and she fell to the floor. I held her up against the window, and then she fell forward. Her being my sister made a great deal of difference—thinking of her as my sister, I stopped—any other person I would have killed. Later on after this a crowd of boys started teasing me about being a crazy veteran. They'd say, "Planes are coming, Duck!" It wasn't too long until I went out of my mind and threatened to kill them.

N–20. Threatened them. [*Restating.*]

P–21. I had a rifle, and I told the bartender in the neighborhood that I was going to kill one. A few days later I went into the hospital as I realized I had lost control of myself.

N–22. Voluntarily. [*Verbalizing the implied for confirmation.*]

P–23. Yes. Most of it was my imagination. They bothered me, but not that much.

N–24. Your imagination? [*Restating to encourage clarification.*]

P–25. Yes, I thought they were being rude to the girl because I wouldn't join the crowd.

N–26. You thought? [*Restating. The nurse is attempting to emphasize the patient's obvious difficulty in distinguishing what is real from his impressions. She may find it helpful to make this observation directly.*]

P–27. Yes, Jane S. I thought she would be my friend. I wrote her letters and told her the crowd should not be rude to her because I wouldn't join. I wrote her these letters, and she didn't like this. My brother went to the door, and she gave my letters back. Some were 18 to 30 pages. Then, I wrote two more, and she wrote a note and said that she would go to far extremes if I didn't stop. I went to a party and tried to talk to her and said her parents had an idea that I was not the right character. Then later one of the boys invited me out, and I almost got involved in a fight. I talked him out of fighting.

Later, I wrote her another letter. I was weakened and under continuous pressure, but I had more to say. My sister told me that the same guy who wanted to fight me came to the house. Then, I made several records and gave them to her. This also made her angry. When I got to the hospital, my sister met her at a bar and grill, and Jane told my sister Mary all the things I had done. She also said to tell him that she was asking for me.

I was bewildered by it and happy, so I wrote her a couple of letters, and she never answered. That crowd made me so miserable, and I'm still upset and my feelings are hurt. I wish that I had never seen them. [*His "hurt feelings" might be explored.*]

N–28. It's time to end the session. [*Giving information. Summarization indicated.*]

(The nurse and patient went to the canteen. He appeared to be less tense than usual. He made a few comments about his sister. He said, "I'll write her a letter and apologize; that's the only thing I can do.")

When the patient states that he imagined or thought certain things, the nurse should help him distinguish reality from fiction by encouraging him to describe what he actually observed. Then he can explore his impressions and their source.

Twenty-eighth Hour

P–1. I thought we'd start off by talking about our trips to the canteen. The third from the last time, when returning, it left me with a blank mind, tense, headache, and sweaty.

N–2. What were your feelings before we went? [*Encouraging description of perceptions.*]

P–3. Don't remember. The next to the last time my brain felt warm and very tired.

N–4. Your brain felt tired. Tell me more so I can follow. [*Exploring. Seeking clarification.*]

P–5. My forehead—pressure and tight skin on my forehead and a slight headache. My head, skin, and ears were moving.

N–6. It felt like the skin on your head was moving? [*Restating. Emphasizing that this was his impression.*]

P–7. I could tell the skin on my head and my ears were moving. I felt mentally weak and couldn't do anything for a couple of hours.

N–8. You had an exhausted feeling? [*Restating for clarification.*]

P–9. An exhausted feeling, yes.

N–10. What were your feelings before we went to the canteen? [*Encouraging description. Placing in sequence. Indicating that there are causes for his anxiety.*]

P–11. I can't remember, but I think I felt okay. Perhaps you have noticed that I can't smile at the end of our sessions. I have been taking aspirin every other day for headaches, and this I think is due to the strain

I put on myself thinking during the interviews. Actually this is expected because I think a lot of things I want to forget. We alleviated the canteen tension by coming right back.

N–12. You like to go to the canteen? [*Encouraging evaluation.*]

P–13. It builds my morale. That is if we go and come right back. Then there's no problem. The next topic I want to talk about is suicide. The first time—or since I was in the Army—I've wanted to kill myself. It never entered my mind before I went into the service.

N–14. What brought on these feelings? [*Placing in sequence. Encouraging description of what preceded this thought.*]

P–15. Before I went into the Army, I was a failure in two businesses. I don't know why, but I got these feelings in the Army. I disliked the Army intensely.

N–16. What things did you dislike? [*Focusing. Encouraging description.*]

P–17. The life of being a soldier. It's a hard life—drills, combat training. I was in the Army two years. When I had to do K.P., I first thought of suicide because I hated doing K.P. so very, very much.

N–18. Just what was it that you disliked in K.P.? [*Encouraging description.*]

P–19. In K.P. I felt like I was being driven to the point where I couldn't be driven—thought that they were working me much too hard. I could never keep up with the inspections, and I was always being gigged.

N–20. Tell me about being gigged. [*Exploring.*]

P–21. The worst thing was the rifle not being clean. They would punish the platoon as a whole—when I did something wrong, they punished everyone—and in basic training, I had no friends—no one liked me.

N–22. What were your feelings about this? [*Reflecting. Encouraging description.*]

P–23. I felt like committing suicide.

N–24. It's hard for me to follow your thinking. [*Seeking clarification.*]

P–25. I was physically exhausted. They would march the hell out of us all day, then bring us back and expect us to have enough strength to pass inspection. In Korea I was so depressed that I didn't care if I got shot. I was worked much too hard. I took every chance to get killed. When I went on patrol, I took a cigarette when it was against the rules.

N–26. What else? [*Offering a general lead. The nurse is aware that if he really wanted to be killed, he must have done more than this.*]

P–27. I was so exhausted that I didn't give my rifle a good cleaning, and there was inspection, and I left a bullet in the rifle.

N–28. Go on. [*Offering a general lead.*]

P–29. Nothing happened to me because I was a medic, and they were kind to me because their life depended on us. In combat the medics carry rifles—he is a rifleman until someone gets hurt, then he takes care of the injured.

N–30. Could you be more specific? [*Encouraging description in greater detail. The nurse might also voice doubt, "Medics carried rifles?"*]

P–31. At points in combat I was weary almost to the point of being delirious.

N–32. At what things? [*Exploring. Perhaps she should use his words, "At what points?"*]

P–33. In times of being physically exhausted. We'd start about 5 P.M., and we'd go into no-man's-land, and we wouldn't get back until about a half hour after dawn. All that time we had to keep our eyes open in case the enemy attacked. I got the feeling as I seen a few men die that if they were killed, it wouldn't make so much difference if I would die, because in comparison my own life seemed less important. [*The nurse might explore: less importance to his life than what?*] I attached less importance to my own life. And when we got back we had breakfast of C rations. Then, we had to work on one project or another—improving the grounds, building latrines, or any kind of work around the camp. This we did until 12 noon; then, we'd eat C rations again. Then we had to clean our rifles and hit the sack. That amounted to about three hours' sleep a day. So you can see I had very little time to rest. But, my problem didn't end there. I had a litter bearer who was extremely nervous and frightened at the idea of going into combat and risking his life, and he used to babble about his wife and kids, and he kept me awake talking about them. He was jittery, nervous, and frightened.

N–34. What were your feelings about this? [*Reflecting.*]

P–35. I wanted to have him transferred to another job. He used to foul up my work. I used to go out on patrols that he was to go out on.

N–36. And. . . . [*Offering a general lead.*]

P–37. Towards the last few days in combat I managed to get him transferred. I was very surprised and disappointed that I wasn't killed in combat.

N–38. Tell me more about this feeling of disappointment. [*Exploring. Encouraging description.*]

P–39. Fifty per cent of the men were lost, and I thought of all the chances that I took—thought I'd get killed too.

N–40. What were some of the chances you took? [*Exploring.*]

P–41. The litter bearer and I were to take turns going out, and I went out three times to his one. I used to smoke cigarettes in the foxhole, and this was serious, and if the enemy saw the light, we'd have trouble—I tried to keep this from the platoon sergeant. [*The nurse might have noted, "This would endanger others as well."*] Another time I was in the foxhole with another soldier, and he said to me that he thought he saw the enemy.

N–42. Go on. [*Offering a general lead.*]

P–43. So he asked me if he should throw a hand grenade, and I said, "Yes." I knew there was no one out there, but I told him to throw the hand grenade.

N–44. Then. . . . [*Offering a general lead.*]

P–45. Then I shot at a branch that was moving in front of us, and in doing this we let the enemy know where we were—this is just another example of how reckless I was. I'm still surprised that I'm still alive. According to the law of averages, I should be dead. Since I've been back home from the Army, I've tried to kill myself eight times—three times by gas, two times by hanging, one time with poison, and two times by slashing my arm.

N–46. Tell me about them. [*Exploring. Encouraging description.*]

P–47. When I took gas, I turned the oven on and stuck my head in the oven for about 15 minutes.

N–48. Then. . . . [*Offering a general lead. She might also ask what led up to each attempt.*]

P–49. I'd get headaches; then I'd stop. I'd do this when my mother and father were on vacation. The slashes—this was two or three years ago —do you want to see them? (Showed his arm.)

N–50. What preceded this? [*Placing in sequence.*]

P–51. I remember that I was demented. [*"Demented" needs clarification.*] At this particular time I didn't have a job, and I wasn't getting along with my parents. At another time I paid $15 to a man for poison. I drank the poison with soda and went to bed. Previous to going to sleep I felt a tingling sensation all over my body and was disappointed the next morning to find that I was still alive.

N–52. What caused the feeling at this time? [*Requesting an explanation. Better worded, "What events took place at this time?" or "What happened before this attempt?"*]

P–53. I was a failure in general—love life, how I was making out with my friends—and I didn't have a girl friend. I didn't get along with my father. I have made plans to drown myself at Shelter Island next. And I plan to make every effort to get a satisfactory poison. I consider myself a failure—not being married—other people consider me a success, but I consider myself a failure.

N–54. You're not feeling so well? [*Verbalizing the implied. The feeling of failure should be explored.*]

P–55. No, it's not that I feel so bad, but down deep I wish I were dead. My people seem to feel that those people who don't get married are bums.

N–56. We covered quite a bit of material; let's summarize. [*Briefly reviewing topics covered.*] We discussed your feeling of being tense when we go to the canteen, your feelings when you had the K.P. assignment in the service, the chances you took when in combat, and the times you tried to commit suicide after returning from the Army. What do you think was learned by the discussion today? [*Encouraging evaluation. The nurse asks too much. Learning requires more than description.*]

P–57. What I learned from this?

N–58. Were there any conclusions? [*Clarifying.*]

P–59. It's not so much what I have learned, but it is a relief to me that through you I know the doctor understands me better. For a couple of months I felt that I wasn't being understood—now I know he'll know.

N–60. After you talk about this, do you feel better? [*Encouraging evaluation. Perhaps better worded, "In what way are your feelings different?"*]

P–61. I feel tired and mentally exhausted. I feel that I'm further understood through you by the doctor, and by thinking about things, I have learned a lot more about myself. Now I realize that I must talk about the problem.

N–62. By working through one problem, you can help yourself think through other problems. [*Giving information about the purpose of the relationship.*]

P–63. Before the interview with you, I did little or no thinking about myself. I never thought of myself as being important enough, and I'm learning a lot about myself that I never knew before.

N–64. We'll continue on Monday. [*Giving information.*]

P–65. Yes, I'd like to talk about my father then.

(The nurse and the patient went to the canteen. The patient talked less than usual. His purchases included coffee, cigarettes, and a newspaper.)

Twenty-ninth Hour

P–1. Hello, I have a lot to tell you today. I have about 35 pages on Jane S. This girl has hurt my feelings more than anyone else in the last four years and second only to my combat experience and in my life. But before I go into this, I want to tell you about my feelings on our last trip to the canteen. These symptoms that I felt. . . .

N–2. Symptoms. . . . [*Restating.*]

P–3. Yes, I felt all the old symptoms coming back, but I was less affected when we came right back. Now, I feel less shaken up. Before we go, I feel mentally exhausted from the interview, but because we went out and came right back, I don't feel it as much as I used to. When I got back, there was the same shifting of the skin on the skull and ears "wiggling," a blankness of mind, and perhaps you didn't see it, but I was slightly rude when you left me at the door of the ward.

N–4. Tell me more so that I can follow what you mean. [*Seeking clarification. Better worded, ". . . so that I can follow what you're saying."*]

P–5. I didn't want to look you in the eye because I had a stiffness of the face.

N–6. I hadn't noticed. [*Presenting reality, indicating that the "stiffness" is not visible.*]

P–7. I thought you didn't. I sense my face expressions are losing a lot of friends for me.

N–8. Tell me more. [*Exploring.*]

P–9. People expect smiles, but I'm not capable of smiling. A couple of years back I wouldn't have been able to smile if Bob Hope were telling jokes.

N–10. What do you think causes this? [*Requesting an explanation. Perhaps the nurse could ask for a description of what does take place. What expressions replace or prevent his smiling and what are his feelings, since smiling is usually an expression of positive feelings.*]

P–11. It's one of the many signs of shock—seeing men die left an indelible effect on me. I saw quite a few men die in Korea. I said "so long" [end of last trip to canteen] a little abruptly and wanted to run to the ward where I'm protected from my gestures. [*What "gestures"?*] I didn't feel like saying goodbyes because I felt a blankness of mind, and I get a little afraid when I do this because I'm afraid I'll do something wrong.

N–12. Such as? [*Offering a general lead.*]

P–13. Lose control of my hands—that I'll scream. I'm afraid that I might elope or run away.

N–14. Did you have any of these feelings lately, particularly when we went to the canteen or here on the ward? [*Exploring.*]

P–15. I've not felt this loss of control when we went out. I just want to keep from losing control.

N–16. Will you tell me when you have these feelings so that we can talk about them? [*Encouraging description of perceptions when they occur.*]

P–17. Yes, I understand and I will. Now we'll continue with Jane S. When she and her girl friends first sat on my stoop, I considered it a strange coincidence that I used to pal around with a soldier with this name in the service. When the crowd was on the stoop, they picked a girl named Marie P. to be my girl friend, but she was extremely nasty to me so I didn't bother with her. It was quite some time before I noticed Jane S.—anyway the crowd was bothering me, and I left home for a year.

N–18. Because of the crowd? [*Verbalizing the implied.*]

P–19. Yes, I go on to explain how the crowd gradually caused me to break down and made me sick. When I came back after a year, I joined the American Legion post and discovered Jane S.'s father was a past post commander. So, it was important for me to have the respect of her mother and father—but it seemed, or maybe I imagined, that her mother and father had negative ideas about me.

N–20. Negative ideas. [*Restating. Focusing on "negative ideas" to encourage description of them.*]

P–21. Yes. One of the ideas was probably that I consorted with kids much younger than I. Of course, this isn't true because they sat on my stoop and likened themselves to me and not me to them. I asked through a messenger to talk to her, and I explained how I thought her mother and father had some wrong impressions of me. I asked her to give her mother and father a truthfully good impression of me.

N–22. A truthfully good impression? [*Restating to bring out more detail.*]

P–23. That I was a gentleman, and I wanted her mother and father to think of me as a gentleman. She didn't say anything, and I walked away thinking that she would surely do this because I see no reason why she shouldn't. She was a very upsetting girl. She seemed to give an invitation to be friendly and then act like you were bothering her. I thought a great deal about the Cool Cats, which is what they called themselves. I tried to attach meaning to their presence and what influence brought them to me. I believe that it was influence from the American Legion post that brought Jane S. to me. You'll notice how my thinking becomes abnormal as we go along—this is the beginning when I started to become deranged. I looked at the crowd in a supernatural way.

N–24. Supernatural way? [*Restating to encourage clarification.*]

P–25. In the sense that the crowd was designed by God.

N–26. Designed by God? [*Restating as a means of seeking clarification.*]

P–27. I believe that there was deep meaning to one's association with people. I imagined that Maureen O. represented my grandmother, because my grandmother I loved deeply, and it left a strong impression on me. Another girl in the crowd I thought represented my mother's strong influence for me. The girl, Marie P., was supposed to be my girl friend, and I believed it because her mother used to date my uncle when they were quite young. She was blond, and my mother told me many years before that I would marry a blond Irish girl. Another girl I thought represented my ambitions away from family influences or the type of girl I would make out with elsewhere was Sue Y. [*His "ambitions away from family influences" would be worth exploring sometime. It is as though he saw himself as a series of parts too diverse to ever become a whole, integrated person.*] Another girl I thought represented my fun-loving type of girl was June Y., her sister. Jane S. was also a blond Irish girl. And I considered her to be the girl I truly rated in life and deserved among the blond Irish girls.

I analyzed from the Cool Cat boys that the Irish in the neighborhood thought well of me. But it seemed to me to be a front because Marie P. had an incurable sickness of the heart. I heard she had only one year to live. I believe the crowd knew this because they wrote it on the walls in the hallway of the apartment house where I used to live and which is my family home. One of the members had the nerve to come bragging to me that they killed her. And the truth is that they certainly helped her into her grave. As you can see, I had a sick outlook but not completely depressing. I didn't wish the crowd to consider me some sort of a snob, so I made efforts to win Marie in front of them all. I proposed marriage to her, and she said "no." I didn't like the crowd and chose not to go too far with them. This proposal showed results of a sick man—that's all I could contribute it to. I showed them that I wanted to cooperate. [*"Wanted to cooperate" is worthy of exploration. He seems to have felt threatened in some way.*] I didn't like the things that they did. I was slowly but surely losing my grip on myself.

I told them that I didn't have time for them and that if the girl was interested, she should sit on my stoop alone or with a girl friend. I seen her alone once in the local ice-cream parlor, and when she saw me, she immediately called her girl friends on the telephone, and she had nothing to say except that she was out drinking with a couple of the boys in the crowd the previous night. She did nothing to show that she was interested in me and seemed to be spiting me by being in the company of bad boys. It was a crowd that had a lot of parties, and they went swimming much during the summer.

When I returned home after Marie died, the crowd didn't have much interest in me, but to show them that in truth I welcomed them but merely didn't like their approach or attitude or goings on, I tried to show a romantic interest in Jane, and that she was in my opinion the girl I respected as being the girl of my soul—trying to explain this was a folly.

N–28. We'll continue next time. [*Giving information. Summarization is definitely indicated. It would be helpful to distinguish just which aspects of the events related he attributes to illness and which aspects are seen as real, and the means by which he distinguishes between the two.*]

Perhaps the nurse can utilize the trips to the canteen to better advantage. Unless she can help him handle the anxiety the trips arouse, it might be better not to go. If, however, he can talk about the pressure on him (to behave in a socially acceptable way in a situation where he is not sure of the rules), it could be most useful. The nurse might say, "You're uncomfortable when you're not certain what's expected of you. It seems unfair, even makes you angry, I imagine. You probably feel annoyed with me for getting you into such a situation." If he can acknowledge these feelings, he may not have to defend against them so vigorously to keep from "losing control."

This nurse-patient relationship was interrupted for a two-week period while the nurse was away for vacation. During their last trip to the canteen, the nurse and the patient discussed what he might do with his time during her absence. The nurse noted, "He agreed to think of the things we've discussed and write down his thoughts and feelings about them."

When the nurse returned, the patient told her that he felt "angry at the hospital, the men, the patients." He stated, "I don't like to talk with you. I think I have gotten worse. Unless we solve the problem how we wish to continue. . . ." When the nurse asked how he wished to continue, he replied, "I suggest that we have more to do with questions. I thought if you asked a couple of questions and I ask some, we could try to solve some of these problems." For the first time the patient seemed to be indicating his readiness to explore his problems with the nurse.

The hour that follows indicates that a new phase in the relationship is evolving, one in which there are both a search for meaning and a beginning collaborative effort.

Thirtieth Hour

P–1. My question is: why can't I drive these crazy thoughts from my mind?

N–2. What are some of your thoughts on this? [*Reflecting.*]

P–3. I get up and walk, and this is the only way I have to shake these thoughts off.

N–4. Would you care to talk about these thoughts? [*Encouraging description.*]

P–5. In combat I got used to hiding myself, and it became deeply instilled in me. When the Cool Cats came in my life, I did the same thing. It's like being trapped. When I get up and walk, it's like a symbol of freedom. When I walk, I stop fearing.

N–6. Tell me about "stop fearing," so I can follow. [*Seeking clarification.*]

P–7. I am afraid of being hurt. Like the Cool Cats—they threatened to beat me up.

N–8. I still have difficulty following what there is to hurt you. [*Seeking clarification.*]

P–9. That shows you where I'm sick.

N–10. Would you tell me more? [*Exploring.*]

P–11. I don't think anything could hurt me here, though I get in difficulty with some of the men. [*"Difficulty with some of the men" should be explored.*]

N–12. What are some of the things you think about which you feel hurt you? [*Encouraging description.*]

P–13. I think about my combat career, and that depresses me. I think about the Cool Cats. I think about the hurt like my sister had, and that depresses me. I think about Frank. It seems I have run into a lot of people I don't like. I am further depressed when I think about my litter bearer in Korea, and my cousin, a fellow named Riley. I got disgusted about a fellow named Parker that I met in combat.

N–14. The main thing is that you're afraid you're going to be hurt? The things we talked about are things that hurt and depress you? [*Summarizing for confirmation. Most appropriate.*]

P–15. Yes.

N–16. Since we have talked about many of these things, have you come to any conclusions? [*Encouraging patient to continue summarizing.*]

P–17. The Cool Cats—I will get over that when I get a new girl friend. About my combat, when I see an Army picture, I cry, and I feel weak, depressed, nervous, and going to pieces. One time something happened. A certain squad leader blamed me because a man was hurt, so I volunteered to go out on the next patrol. He insulted my courage, and I wanted to show him that I was brave. Then I couldn't go because the officer stopped me and said, "See Old Paint. You can go out tomorrow night." My father once said people get bad habits much quicker than they get good habits. Maybe that's the answer to this situation. If I get a girl friend, it would overcrowd these memories. Girls have a tremendous influence on a man. Life to me is a psychological trap. Say, why can't we go to the canteen alone?

N–18. It's the doctor's order that one of the aides go with us. [*Giving information. Making limits known.*]

P–19. I gave away my money today.

N–20. You didn't want it? [*Seeking clarification.*]

P–21. I need the money.

N–22. What were you trying to buy? [*Exploring.*]

P–23. I don't know. Maybe I was trying to buy friends.

N–24. Do you think you can buy friendship? [*Reflecting.*]

P–25. Yes, in one way or another, but not true friends.

N–26. So what is your conclusion about giving money away for this purpose? [*Encouraging summarization.*]

P–27. I'm disgusted with myself. And since I gave it away, I have a pain in my hip. Then, too, in the process I hoped I was trying to buy a friend.

N–28. Aren't there other ways to gain friendship? [*Introducing related aspect of the topic.*]

P–29. I don't know. There's a cold situation here. I don't think I have a friend on the ward.

N–30. Just being yourself many times gains friends. Last time I was here, one of the patients came to me and introduced himself as one of your friends, and on other occasions when we went to the canteen, various people stopped and spoke to you in a friendly manner. [*Giving information in an area in which this patient is sorely lacking. Recalling previous observations.*]

P–31. But I'm displeased with the things I say and do. Sometimes I'm a totally difficult character.

N–32. Do you ever think of your good qualities? [*Introducing related aspect of topic.*]

P–33. Yes, I'm thankful for not being without an arm or leg—that I'm reasonably attractive.

N–34. Think about these qualities, and we can talk about them at another time. [*Encouraging further evaluation.*]

P–35. In combat, my litter bearer—I thought he felt I was going to kill him because he was German.

N–35. What gave you this impression? [*Encouraging description of perceptions.*]

P–37. He always seemed nervous when I was around.

P–38. Now I'll have more questions for you next time. Can we go to the canteen now?

(The nurse and patient went to the canteen.)

The hour ended, but the relationship goes on. How long it will need to continue cannot be predetermined. But much is yet to be accomplished. The patient is just beginning to try to understand his problems in relating to others and to see the nurse as an active collaborator rather than as a passive listener.

Study 17. *MR. ALBERT S.*______

A Relationship with a Patient on a Disturbed Unit

The patient, aged 36, was one of four male siblings of a household with many domestic problems. A frequent truant, he completed only two years of high school before he was asked to leave because of being "asocial and rebellious." At 16, he joined the Merchant Marine under his brother's name. He later entered the military service during World War II. In 1954 the patient started drinking heavily, reportedly because of his brother's death. He was admitted to the hospital in 1961 because he had become delusional, expressing bizarre religious ideas. The nurse-patient relationship started three weeks after admission and four days after he had torn down marble bathroom partitions, throwing them at personnel. This behavior followed the denial of his request to have his blood drained to prove that he was Christ and could not die.

First Day

N–1. Good morning, Al. [*Expressing recognition. The patient's proper name, Mr. S., would be more appropriate.*]

P–2. Good morning, Mr. ____.

(The nurse asked the patient if he could have a little of his time and suggested they sit on the porch. The patient was told that they would be getting together frequently just to talk, also that the nurse would be writing the comments during the conversation. The patient was polite and agreeable to the plan.)

N–3. How is everything going with you? [*The nurse attempted to give the patient an opportunity to state his feelings.*]

P–4. Fine. I feel much more relaxed now.

N–5. How did you feel before? [*Encouraging comparison.*]

P–6. Betrayed.

N–7. Why would you feel betrayed? [*Exploring. Requesting an explanation.*]

P–8. I went off the deep end. (The patient appeared to have difficulty remembering.)

N–9. What did the nurse say to you? [*Introducing an unrelated topic.*]

P–10. It's clear now. My request to the staff was unacceptable.

N–11. What was your request? [*Seeking clarification.*]

P–12. To draw all the blood out of me. Too much mysterious . . . happening to me. I am Jesus Christ and by draining my blood will prove to the world that what I say is so.

N–13. When did you first begin to have these ideas? [*Attempting to place in sequence. The nurse is attempting to place the event in its historical perspective.*]

P–14. I had been in Kansas City for a plumbers' convention. I was under a great deal of strain. I did plenty of drinking but no women. As I was crossing the street one morning. . . .

N–15. What time? [*The nurse has interrupted the patient by attempting to focus on a minor detail.*]

P–16. About 10 in the morning. A bolt of lightning struck between my legs. I went to my room and heard "Glory, Glory, Hallelujah" sung by a choir. I wondered if I had the D.T.'s and made a vow never to drink again.

N–17. What happened when you left Kansas City? [*The nurse has moved the discussion of events ahead in time.*]

P–18. I got the urge to look at the Bible. The numbers 6 to 69 pertained to the return of Christ. The priest was very anxious to get me in here.

N–19. Why? [*Requesting an explanation. The nurse is attempting to clarify an idea. The use of the word "why" requires the patient to give reasons for his thoughts when the objective should be to have the patient describe these ideas.*]

P–20. He was afraid I would scare a lot of people and for my own protection.

N–21. Why do you think we have these types of hospitals? [*Testing the patient's insight.*]

P–22. For people with mental problems. I was going to ask my wife why the priest. . . . (Interrupted by another patient who spoke to the nurse saying, "This S.O.B. has come to me as the devil.") He can't stare me in the eye, can you? (The second patient answered, "I can stare you in the eye in the dark! That proves I'm the devil.") You know that man on the other ward with the beard is Moses, and he was following the doctor when I was sent here. [*It would have been meaningful for the nurse to find out what this meant to the patient.*]

N–23. Do you think you have a mental problem? [*The nurse has changed the subject and is testing the patient's insight.*]

P–24. I don't think I have. I missed the boat on the whole answer—whether I am Jesus Christ. When I returned from Kansas City I went to Dr. ____ to see about my problem. My wife suggested I see a priest. Dr. ____ recommended hospitalization for a few days' observation. I did! Did I tell you what I did with my glasses? I tried to kill myself which I couldn't do and to prove what I am.

N–25. What did you prove? [*The patient has admitted having a problem, and the nurse has failed to explore this lead. Challenging. As a result, the patient may be forced to strengthen and expand his misinterpretations of reality by seeking support for his point of view.*]

P–26. Something is miraculous.

N–27. Has treatment helped you any? [*Asking the patient to evaluate his treatment.*]

P–28. Hasn't changed the thought processes—has calmed me down—not as jumpy as hell as when I came here. I thought I was being sold down the river as Christ was by Judas. If you read the new version, it sets my mind at ease. It says the numbers can be found by man. When I returned from Kansas City, these numbers came off my driver's license—too many 6s and 69s coming into my life.

N–29. Why do you feel like that patient belongs here rather than you? [*The nurse has changed the topic of conversation by introducing an unrelated topic. The patient's insight is again being tested.*]

P–30. He drinks water all day and sits in the "john." Patient ____ doesn't belong here either. I dislike patient ____. Patient ____ is the angel of death.

N–31. What makes you say that? [*The nurse has used a negative approach in an attempt to clarify a point. The existence of an external source is being indicated.*]

P–32. The way he arose from his bed. I am going to see what my wife is doing about my revelations. I assume she is letting people know I am in this hospital, but I want them to know why.

(This was the end of the first meeting.)

Second Day

N–1. Good morning, Al.

P–2. So what happens now! The doctors have looked me over.

N–3. What did they look you over for? [*The nurse is again testing the patient's insight.*]

P–4. They thought I was hitting the bottle.

N–5. Which doctors came to see you? [*Seeking clarification.*]

P–6. Drs. _____, _____, and _____.

N–7. How was your visit with your wife? [*Introducing an unrelated topic.*]

P–8. Very nice.

N–9. How is she doing? [*The patient is obviously having many problems of his own. The nurse is asking him to evaluate his wife's situation when he is not ready to evaluate his own.*]

P–10. Struggling along without me. (Smiling.)

N–11. Does she work? [*The nurse is pursuing more detail on the patient's wife's situation.*]

P–12. She takes care of one little house. She's applying for compensation. I'd like to see the clay drop from my feet next week.

N–13. Do you think you're ready? [*The patient is asked to evaluate his own condition.*]

P–14. Sure, I'm ready. I don't belong here.

(The patient and the nurse sat looking about the dayroom. The patient did not appear to be occupied with anything in particular. His face had a rather blank and uninspired expression.) [*During such periods of silence, it is important that the nurse is aware of his own expressions. Silence can encourage the patient to verbalize if it is an interested and expectant silence. It gives the patient an opportunity to collect and organize his thoughts, to think through a point, or to consider introducing a topic of greater concern.*]

P–15. How many patients in this hospital?

N–16. Twenty-five hundred, give or take a few. [*Giving information. However, the patient has reversed roles and is interviewing the nurse.*]

P–17. When did they start here?

N–18. About 1929. [*Giving information.*]

P–19. I used to be around here when I was a kid with my father. We used to visit my uncle. (Conversation interrupted by another patient requesting a light—followed by a period of silence.) If you could have seen it as I saw it, you'd flip. (Referring to the patient he describes as the angel of death.)

N–20. How do you get along with the other patients? [*Introducing an unrelated topic. The nurse has ignored the patient's lead.*]

P–21. All right. Everyone wants to shake my hand and not slap me. Right ____? (The patient was seeking confirmation from another patient. The second patient was openly hostile and threatening. The first patient looked at the nurse, shrugged his shoulders, and smiled.)

N–22. What are your plans? [*The nurse is testing the patient's ability to plan the future.*]

P–23. I'm going back to plumbing. I was working right here in ____ on that new school. I was a foreman on that job. (Hesitated. Banged cast.) I'll be loused up for a couple of weeks with this damn thing. (Silence.) Did you see the shiner ____ has?

N–24. Who did it? [*The nurse is seeking information about a ward incident.*]

P–25. Mr. ____.

N–26. When did it happen? [*Seeking information. The discussion is no longer focused on the patient. Each hour seems to end without preparation or closing comments.*]

Third Day

(The patient had been notified that certification proceedings had been instituted.)

N–1. Hello, Al.

P–2. I have more faith in the justice of the United States. How can they let this happen? How can my wife make a petition?

N–3. Your wife, being the nearest of kin, is legally responsible for your actions. This is most likely a routine using her name due to her relationship. [*The nurse is giving a somewhat evasive explanation of this very important proceeding.*]

P–4. That's true, but I wonder if she knows about this. I'll bet she doesn't. Something like this just doesn't happen in the United States. When is the 16th? I want to call my wife.

N–5. We'd have to get permission for you to call. [*Stating restriction. Permission from whom?*]

P–6. Why? I called when I was on Ward ____.

N–7. Well, it's not a regular thing to have the patient use the phones, and each doctor must give his approval. [*The nurse has explained the restriction mentioned.*]

P–8. Well, don't bother asking Dr. ____ because he doesn't like me anyway.

N–9. What makes you say that? [*Seeking clarification in a negative manner, implying that the source is external to the patient.*]

P–10. Well, this morning when he was making rounds, I asked him what recourse I had to get out of here. He told me I would have to stay until I was better. Where's Dr. ____?

N–11. Dr. ____ is off today but should be back tomorrow. [*Giving information.*]

P-12. Who's paying for these physicians to examine me? Me? Can I call my wife? I know she knows nothing about this.

N–13. All I can do is ask Dr. ____ if he will give permission. [*The nurse is explaining his own limitations.*]

P–14. He won't, but you can try. I'm being railroaded. I have no recourse. I want legal representation. You people can't hold me now. I'll be there.

N–15. Why don't you wait until visiting day when your wife will be here? You can ask her all about this at that time. You can also make arrangements for legal representation if you still want it. [*The nurse is offering the patient a course of action; however, the wife will bear the brunt of his hostile feelings.*]

P–16. She won't have time.

N–17. There'll be plenty of time. At least four days. [*Giving information.*]

Fourth Day

N–1. Hello, Al.

P–2. Have you seen Mr. ____? [A newly admitted patient.]

N–3. Yes, I saw him when he arrived. [*Giving information.*]

P–4. Do you know who he is?

N–5. Yes, I told you. [*The nurse is acknowledging another patient.*]

P–6. He's God Almighty in disguise, and the Day of Judgment will be held in the courtyard.

N–7. I notice he has a cauliflower ear. [*The nurse has unknowingly disagreed with the patient in a subtle manner. The patient is apparently delusional, and the nurse has noted a reality factor that does not fit.*]

P–8. That's a disguise. Do you know who these guys are in the trucks outside fixing the road?

N–9. No. They appear to be workmen. [*The nurse appears to be uncertain as to their identity. If their identity were known, it should have been stated as fact.*]

P–10. They're the angels of God, and they're all ex-marines. They're here to look out for the veterans.

N–11. Why would they be fixing the roads? [*Seeking clarification. Requesting an explanation.*]

P–12. Because when Judgment Day arrives, there's going to be a lot of cars leaving here and going mighty fast. You don't believe me?

N–13. It's hard to see these people as you do, Al. To me they appear as an old man who is sick and needs help. The workmen appear as workmen, none of whom I know, and whose military history is a mystery to me. [*The nurse has presented his own evaluation of the persons the patient has misidentified. However, he has ended poorly by stating "whose military history is a mystery to me." This somewhat supports the patient's delusional ideation that something is mysterious about the goings on about the hospital.*]

P–14. Mark my words, L., the Day of Judgment is coming, and it will be in the courtyard. God help everyone.

Fifth Day

N–1. Good morning, Al.

(The patient arose from his wheelchair and walked with a full leg cast.)

N–2. Sit down, Al. [*The nurse has given a direct command.*]

P–3. I don't need this. (Banging cast.) My bones are healed. God has arrived and I am cured. He told me so.

N–4. You better make sure that it is healed before you walk too much on it. [*Advising.*]

P–5. It's for sure I'm healed.

N–6. I'll have to go now, Al. [*The nurse's departure appears hasty.*]

P–7. Don't forget to see Mr. _____. He's God Almighty.

The nurse has not been too successful in his attempts to develop a therapeutic nurse-patient relationship. The patient needs to know that the nurse is interested in him as a person, that he is interested in his feelings and ideas. It is necessary for the patient to know this, and he can be told this outright. The nurse should tell the patient that he can talk to him about anything he wants. By doing this, the initiative is left up to the patient.

The nurse should ask questions primarily when it is necessary to get the patient to describe more fully what he brings up. At the second and third meetings, the patient did not mention his delusional ideas. This was possibly a result of the reluctance of the nurse to discuss them. The relationship between the nurse and the patient up to this point appears to be a superficial one.

Sixth Day

N–1. How are things, Al? [*Giving the patient a broad opening. A rather stereotyped expression, however.*]

P–2. Same old nonsense, I don't know why the hell I'm still here. I don't know why I came here from the other ward.

N–3. You must have been upset for them to send you here. I think you mentioned someone being responsible for your being here. [*Giving information about his transfer to a disturbed ward. The word "them" should be avoided, and the nurse should be specific. Patients refer too often to vaguely defined other persons as "they."*]

P–4. Mr. _____. No, he didn't have anything to do with it. (Silence.) Today's the day they commit me.

N–5. Did you talk to your wife about it? [*Asking for information.*]

P–6. Yes. She didn't know anything about it. Dr. _____ said they can't do anything about it.

N–7. Have you been receiving treatments? [*Introducing a new topic. If the nurse did not know, the question is warranted. However, if the nurse already knows that the patient is receiving treatment, he is testing. If it is the nurse's intent to learn how the patient feels about the treatments, he should ask directly.*]

P–8. What are they supposed to do for me?

N–9. They should help you relax. [*The nurse has given only a partial explanation of the treatment.*]

P–10. I'm relaxed, but I can blow off at a drop of a pin. I've shown I can control my temper, haven't I?

N–11. Yes. You appear to be more accepting of your hospitalization. [*The nurse is telling the patient that he is being cooperative or "good." If the nurse thinks that the patient is controlling the expression of his feelings, he should say so. Stating that the patient is accepting his hospitalization is an indication to him that the nurse does not understand him. The nurse might better have described his behavior as calmer.*]

N–12. If you can still blow off at a drop of a pin, you must still need help. [*The patient may be maintaining his control with difficulty, and it might be better to ask him what it is that upsets him.*]

P–13. I don't need help. I should be home with my wife and kids. Look, I can get myself a good union job as a business agent.

N–14. I'll bet it has a lot of social-activity requirements. [*The nurse appears to be trying to have the patient admit he has a problem with alcohol and that he will have a difficult time solving this problem. The nurse should consider whether alcohol has been used, unsuccessfully, as a solution to more basic problems.*]

P–15. Yes, but I'm not going to drink any more.

N–16. How can you say that? [*Expressing disbelief.*]

P–17. Because I know.

N–18. You've been drinking a good many years, and it's something you just don't stop. [*Disagreeing.*]

P–19. I know I won't.

N–20. Listen! Do you think you'll ask for water when you're hooking up pipe? [*Expressing disbelief.*]

P–21. You're right, but the way I feel now I don't have to drink again.

N–22. How do you feel? [*Seeking clarification. Better worded, "What are your feelings now?"*]

P–23. Somewhat calmer, but I want to get out.

Seventh Day

N–1. Good morning.

P–2. Good morning, Mr. L.
(Silence. The patient appeared very solemn. He arose from his chair and walked to the bathroom.)

N–3. If that leg of yours heals, it will be amazing. [*Expressing disapproval.*]
(Silence.)

Eighth Day

N–1. Hi, Al.

P–2. Mr. L. How's things?

N–3. Sounds like you have a cold, too. [*The nurse indicates that she* *notices the patient's physical condition. Making such observations develops the feeling of interest in the patient.*]

P–4. Right, only slight. It's been on and off for the past two weeks.

N–5. What are you taking for it? [*The nurse is continuing to show interest in the care the patient is receiving.*]

P–6. Aspirin.

N–7. Did you have any visitors? [*The nurse has introduced a topic for conversation. However, it is suggested that the patient be given the opportunity to introduce the topic.*]

P–8. Yes, with my wife, son, and daughter. My wife loves me very much, and my children miss me. I live at 16 ____ ____ and I'm married to ____. My son was here with his wife.

N–9. With your wife? [*Seeking clarification. The nurse should be prepared to do this whenever there is any doubt as to what has been said. It is essential that both participants understand each other.*]

P–10. With his wife. He's 21 years old and from my wife's first marriage. I adopted him. I have two children by this marriage. Both boys. My wife just bought the younger boy a bike.

N–11. What school do they go to? [*The nurse is again seeking information of an apparently irrelevant nature.*]

P–12. They both go to public school. One's in the second grade and the other's in the sixth.

N–13. Would you send them to parochial school? [*Seeking information. The nurse has a purpose in asking the question; however, it may not have been apparent to the patient. If there is a purpose for gaining further information, the nurse should explain it. Otherwise, the patient may have good reason for becoming suspicious.*]

P–14. Yes, but there are none around.

N–15. Did you go to parochial school? [*The nurse appears to be taking an interviewer's approach. The patient's past experiences should come out naturally as he wants to discuss them. This type of question will obtain facts but little information about the patient's feelings.*]

P–16. Yes, but we were put out. I was put out with my older brother. He got in trouble, and they figured I would be bothersome too; so out we went. This school was in ____ and you have to have it or else you don't belong.

N–17. What kind of work do your brothers do? [*The nurse is seeking more information but broadening the scope of the subject instead of focusing on one phase of it.*]

P–18. They're all plumbers. One brother was killed in Virginia. We make about five and a quarter an hour. I've lost about a $1000 since I've been here.

N–19. Your health is more important. [*The nurse is preaching and possibly challenging the patient to defend himself and his state of health.*]

P–20. There's nothing wrong with my health (hesitated), in my estimation anyway. I'll take a sanity test.

N–21. Do you still see other patients as the devil and angels of death? What of the ideas you expressed? [*Testing the patient.*]

P–22. I have those in abeyance.

N–23. Why keep them in abeyance? [*Seeking clarification. The patient is keeping his ideas in abeyance because they are not acceptable to the nurse and, most likely, to others. He expresses this by his response.*]

P–24. You people say they're not true, but if you could see the Sacred Heart floating across the ceiling when I was in hydro' room. If I see them again, I'll know they're true.

N–25. Tell me more about the Sacred Heart. [*The nurse is seeking more detail concerning the patient's comment. It is important to do this so that the patient feels he is not being rejected before the nurse knows what the ideas are and why he believes them.*]

P–26. I was laying in the hydro' room, and the Sacred Heart floated over the ceiling. This was not my imagination.

N–27. Do you still think that Mr. ____ is God Almighty? [*Testing.*]

P–28. Sure he is.

N–29. Well, tell me about it. [*The response to the patient's comment is appropriate. However, the nurse has changed the subject and introduced another.*]

P–30. I saw him in a dream. It's difficult to describe. (Pause.) Let me think—mental block. I know it was a dream.

N–31. Can't you remember? [*Challenging.*]

P–32. I can't remember clearly the dream, but that was where I first met him.

N–33. It seems that if this was so firm in your mind and you were so sure, it should be fairly easy to describe it. Is there anything else you can tell me about Mr. ____, because I don't see him as you do, and I would like you to tell me when all of this came about? [*The nurse is disapproving of the patient's misidentification. The patient is being asked for more details but is also being told that his explanations will be unacceptable. It is desirable to inform the patient that the nurse does not see things as he does. However, this must be done at the opportune time. The development of a good nurse-patient relationship makes minor errors less disastrous.*]

P–34. It all started in Kansas City when I was at the convention. The bolt of lightning struck between my legs and the music in my room. That was the beginning.

N–35. Well, Al, from all reports there wasn't any real storm out that way. [*The nurse is attempting to present reality. In doing so, it is necessary to be factual. "From all reports" is quite vague.*]

P–36. Oh, yes, there was. There was a severe lightning and thunder storm. Those voices singing the hymn.

N–37. Was there a radio in your room? [*The nurse's comment is realistic enough and gives the patient an alternative to consider.*]

P–38. No radio.

N–39. Are you sure you heard these voices? [*Testing. It is important for the nurse to understand the realism of the voices in hallucinations.*]

P–40. They were there, I swear. (Pause.)

N–41. You said you had been drinking a long while, but what made you increase the amount lately? [*Introducing an unrelated topic.*]

P–42. Job pressure. I'm not going to be a foreman any longer. I can't work with my boss. He's too much of a pusher.

N–43. How long have you worked with him? [*Seeking more detail.*]

P–44. Two years, but I can't continue. It's not worth it. He drives people too hard, and I can't work like that.

N–45. Sorry, Al, but I must leave now. I'd like to continue the discussion when we meet again. [*The patient's relationship with his boss is worth exploring further. If the boss expected too much or was overcritical, the patient may have developed a great deal of anxiety in his dealings with him.*]

P–46. Okay. See you!

Ninth Day

N–1. And how are you? [*Asking stereotyped question.*]

P–2. I feel fine. When does this come off? [Referring to his cast.]

N–3. From six to eight weeks. [*The nurse is giving information in a very vague way. The patient should be told what factors determine the removal of the cast.*]

P–4. Well, it's six weeks now, and it's all healed. It was put on September 15th.

N–5. What would you like to talk about? [*The nurse is permitting the* *patient to choose the topic of discussion for the first time. Doing this often indicates an interest in what the patient would like to discuss.*]

P–6. About going home. When am I getting the hell out of here? I'd like to be staffed at the next staff on Thursday. When will Dr. ____ be back?

N–7. I don't know, but I can find out easy enough. How do you think you would impress the staff? [*Testing.*]

P–8. How do you think I'd do?

N–9. I think you'd make a good impression considering how you've improved. [*The nurse is offering an opinion which proves to be misleading by virtue of the patient's response.*]

P–10. They're interested in other things. Why don't you loan me your keys, and let me prove how much better I am?

N–11. You know I'd be fired if I made such a bargain. [*This was the nurse's opportunity to tell the patient that he wants to help him. However, the response implies that the nurse will not let him out because he would get in trouble.*]

P–12. What are some of the better wards around here?

N–13. They're all good, but you wouldn't be able to move until your cast comes off and you can get around by yourself. [*Reassuring. Giving information.*]

N–14. What are you thinking about? [*The patient is being given an opening to discuss his thoughts if he so desires.*]

P–15. I better get myself a good lawyer to prove my sanity. (Pensive.)

N–16. Why don't you describe things as you see them now, Al? [*The nurse is reinforcing his interest in having the patient discuss what is important to him.*]

P–17. Shock has me all screwed up. I don't know what I'm thinking any more.

N–18. What's so confusing? [*Seeking clarification.*]

P–19. Who am I?

N–20. You try and tell me who you are. [*Reflecting. The nurse has made an appropriate comment. The patient's point of view is being sought.*]

P–21. I'm Al S. I live at 16 ____ ____. My wife's name is ____ and I have two children.

N–22. Who do you want to be? [*The nurse continues to give the patient an opportunity to express himself.*]

P–23. Al S. Has shock done this to me? What do you think?

N–24. I think the treatment has helped you feel more like yourself.

[*The nurse has offered his opinion.*] Do you see the other man as you did before? [*Testing.*]

P–25. No.

N–26. How about Mr. ____? [*The nurse is expecting too much from the patient. He is being pressured into denying the existence of past delusional experiences. The nurse might better have pursued the kind of Al S. he wants to be and what he wants for himself.*]

P–27. I must see him before I can say.

N–28. Why must you see him before you can tell whether he's God or not? [*Seeking clarification. Requesting an explanation.*]

P–29. Isn't it possible for Christ to come down to live with His people?

N–30. It may be possible, but if it were to happen why would He come in the form of Mr. ____ and not as He really is? Also wouldn't He be of such a nature that everyone would know who He is and not just yourself? [*Challenging. The most appropriate response to the patient's comment would have been a direct "I don't know." The nurse must be ready to admit this lack of information when it is indicated. The nurse is trying to reason away the patient's delusions.*]

(Pause.)

P–31. Check his service record.

N–32. You're not answering my question. [*The nurse is pressing the patient for a reply.*]

P–33. Check his service record. He was a marine.

N–34. What has that got to do with my question? I'll check his service record if you like, but I know he was a marine. [*Seeking clarification. Offering to comply. Giving information.*]

P–35. How do you know?

N–36. He told me he was, and also I heard him giving close-order drill commands as we used to do. [*Giving explanation, but this is hardly proof.*]

P–37. ____ is all Marine.

N–38. Listen, Al, it's time for me to go. I'd like to go over your Bible with you and for you to show me the passages that lead you to believe as you do about Mr. ____. So long. [*Giving information. Further challenging the patient to "prove" his ideas.*]

The nurse's closing comments were poorly timed. The patient is expressing some doubt or confusion about his own identity. He has implied that maybe he is not Christ and that possibly Mr. ____ is not God. The nurse is asking the patient to support the ideas he is now questioning. It is to be expected that the patient will express the same delusional ideas from time to time. It is hoped that as the relationship continues he will be able to reject them and be himself. When this occurs, he will no longer need to misidentify in order to feel accepted.

The nurse is moving toward a productive nurse-patient relationship as his responses are permitting the patient to express his feelings about topics that are of concern to him. Exploration of delusional ideas should be done, but only when the patient introduces and expresses them. The more the patient is pushed to give them up, the more he may feel he needs them.

Tenth Day

N–1. Good morning, Al. [*Recognition of the patient as a person.*]

P–2. Weird happenings today. It's All Saints' Day. There are two new guys that haven't eaten a thing. They have the evil eye and are devils.

N–3. Bill ____ was a devil, wasn't he? [*Introducing previously expressed delusional ideas. The nurse is attempting to clarify the patient's statement by comparing it with past statements. To explore the patient's idea of "weird happenings" and in what way he considers them "weird" would have been more appropriate.*]

P–4. He straightened himself out.

N–5. "Devil" is a temporary state. [*Verbalizing the implied. The nurse indicates his grasp of what the patient is saying. In addition, the idea of possible change has been opened for discussion.*]

P–6. God gave us confession to absolve our sins.

N–7. I didn't think the devil ever became absolved of his sins and changed. [*The nurse is taking the patient literally. The patient seems to mean "some of the devil" (evil) in them. As a result, he is being lead back to his interpretation of the Bible rather than toward reality.*]

P–8. In final judgment, Lucifer is so sick and tired of sinning, he wants repentance for his sins. He comes back to the Lord. Fresh boys take over and get fresh crew.

N–9. From where? [*Seeking clarification.*]

P–10. From here. I don't know whether I saw C. or not, but they cannot look me in the eye. There's a battle of wills. What has happened is that there is a war going on in heaven with all the angels. They're putting things in the hands of the Virgin Mary. She is going to decide who is going to rule heaven. I wish you'd take an x-ray of my chest to see if I have a ball-point pen in my chest. Tomorrow's All Souls' Day. It's going to be something.

N–11. What's going to happen? [*The nurse's question implies that the patient is able to foretell the future.*]

P–12. (Interrupting.) Beautiful sunrise today.

N–13. What is going to happen tomorrow? [*The nurse continues to persist and is obviously being ignored by the patient.*]

P–14. He's a black-hearted angel. (The patient turned to another patient in the vicinity.) I see light from your eyes; they're trying to corrupt your morals. Those black-hearted sinners. (During this exchange, he was looking into the sun.)

N–15. When you say you saw C., what do you mean? [*The nurse is changing the topic of discussion and digressing to a topic gone by. It must be remembered that the topic of discussion is to be initiated by the patient. When the nurse finds that he has missed an opportunity to explore a comment further, he must wait for his next chance.*]

P–16. I saw his face in the shape of a devil.

N–17. Is he one of the two people? [*Seeking clarification.*]

P–18. No. He's under their control. He's afraid they're going to cut his penis off. He's another one. (Pointing to another patient.) You listening to those black devils? (Speaking to the patient. Another patient approached and said, "Why do we have to be with them or like them?" The patient continued in this manner, identifying different patients present as the heads of the principal churches. Pointing to another patient.) He asked me if he could come to Catholic services. I said "yes."

N–19. Why did he ask you? [*The implication of this comment is a challenge, asking the patient whether he still thinks he is Christ.*]

P–20. I must be the angel of the Catholic Church.

N–21. Do you think you are? [*Reflecting. Challenging. The patient is being placed in an uncomfortable position as he is being pressed to commit himself.*]

P–22. I think it's very possible. I'd love to go to Catholic church.

N–23. At our last meeting you mentioned having all these ideas in abeyance. [*It is difficult to determine what the nurse had in mind when making this comment. If it was intended to find out why the patient can put these ideas aside sometimes and not others, the nurse should have been direct.*]

P–24. What do you mean abeyance?

N–25. That's the word you used. [*Trying to clarify what the word means to the patient. Patients often use words to mean something other than their literal meanings. The patient has avoided further discussion of the word. It is important to keep the patient focused on one idea until it is understood by both participants. This is an important consideration in developing a nurse-patient relationship, since it is vital to communication.*]

P–26. When I look at them, it's a battle of wills.

N–27. Between whom? [*Seeking clarification.*]

P–28. All angels.

N–29. What do you see in the sun? [*Introducing an unrelated topic. Implying that there is something to be seen.*]

P–30. Blessed Virgin Mary.

N–31. Why can you see her and I can't? [*Requesting an explanation. Indicating to the patient that his experiences are different from those of others. However, this might have been noted without the use of "why."*]

P–32. I believe I'm Jesus. All Souls' Day is tomorrow, and something will tell. I think the visitation will be tomorrow. (Looking to the sun and speaking to it.) Will the Resurrection be tomorrow? Please let the Resurrection be tomorrow.

N–33. Did they answer? [*Giving a literal response. The nurse is confronting the patient with the fact that he does not share his experience. However, the word "they" should have been avoided. The nurse might find it valuable to know why the patient wants the Resurrection to occur the next day. He may be tiring of being Christ and desiring an end to his anxiety.*]

(The patient continued to look into the sun and move his lips.)

N–34. Well, Al, are they answering? [*Pressing for an answer.*]

P–35. All I'm doing is praying. [*The patient's reply is an interesting one. The prior comment by the nurse suggested the possibility of auditory hallucinations. The patient is denying this experience. The nurse might better have said, "Will you get an answer?" and avoided the implication.*]

N–36. When the sun comes from behind the clouds, what happens? [*The nurse has remained within the topic of conversation but has not gotten an answer to the question before. The nurse seems to be participating in—even adding to—the patient's delusional thinking.*]

P–37. I get some power from it. (A patient approached.) You're fooling with evil, T. J. is evil and part of the crew. So is P. [*This comment is worth pursuing since it implies a need. It may be significant to know what kind of power he gets and what it is needed for. The patient may feel he, in himself, is powerless to deal with something, such as sin or evil-doing of some sort, or powerless to deal with people in some way. The delusions experienced are not vague, abstract ideas but are of great meaning to the patient. When it is determined what purpose they serve, the nurse may better help him not need them. As has been mentioned, the nurse must wait for openings—for clues—and follow them, without putting words in the patient's mouth.*]

N–38. You said the treatment made you confused. Are you still? [*Introducing an unrelated topic. Testing.*]

P–39. No, everything is clear to me. (Exhibiting Bible.) It's all in here. If you want to take it to read, you can.

N–40. Show me these passages with the numbers 6 and 69. [*Seeking clarification of previous comments made by the patient.*]

N–41. Well, Al, what did you find? [*Pressing.*]

P–42. I have to give you the number.

N–43. No. You don't have to. This is what you base your thoughts on. You were saying to me. . . . [*Challenging.*]

P–44. Long ago, I told you fires were going to fall. Here, read the Bible. When can you get the priest here?

N–45. I'll call and find out. [*Giving assurance of action.*]

P–46. You can't sin more. Repent.

Eleventh Day

N–1. Hi, Al. How're things? [*Giving recognition. Asking stereotyped question.*]

P–2. Fine. Much better. The power play with saints is still on. You have to read this book. Take it with you.

N–3. I'm not a very fast reader; so I'll need it for some time. [*The nurse is suggesting the possibility of his seeing things as the patient does. It would have been better to determine whether this is what the patient had in mind. If it were, the nurse might truthfully have said that it would not be likely.*]

P–4. Let's get down to brass tacks.

N–5. Okay. Let's go. [*The patient has suggested that he wants to talk of matters that are important to him, and the nurse has given him encouragement.*]

P–6. Well, we're all descendants from two people—Adam and Eve.

N–7. Right. [*Agreeing. It would have been sufficient to say, "Go on."*]

P–8. Over the years, the saints got tired of heaven and came to earth in different bodies.

N–9. Why would anyone get tired of heaven and come to earth in a different body? [*Seeking clarification. Requesting an explanation.*]

P–10. Better explained in here than I can explain to you. This man is one of them. (Leafing through the Bible.) Eyes are flashing; I can't read.

N–11. How long has this been going on? [*Placing event in time.*]

P–12. Ever since the revelation came to me. The Lord got His angels and made them equal to Him. The angels became perverted, and that's when war broke out in heaven.

N–13. You're telling me about a story you read, but how do you fit into this picture? [*The nurse is attempting to understand how all this applies to him.*]

P–14. I'm the Lamb of God. These perverts are cast out of heaven and roam the earth. They join the Army, and what's the best country? U.S.A. So they join the Army and live off the government. I asked for my release. I asked to go home to my wife and kids. These are angels. D. is the Lord, and he will save me. What time is it?

N–15. 10:30. [*Giving information.*]

P–16. The sun is bright. (Looking up in silence.) I can look at you without a loss of color. Jesus, I want to go home to my wife and kids. They gave you the evil eye.

N–17. How do they give you the evil eye? [*Seeking clarification. It is important for the nurse to understand what the patient means. His statement "I can look at you without a loss of color" should be explored. Otherwise, the patient is given the impression that the nurse understands when he does not. It is also important to determine who the patient means when he uses words such as "they," "them," "we," "us."*]

P–18. Because I am dangerous. That must be it.

N–19. Are they afraid of you? [*The reflected feeling is appropriate. However, the word "they" should be avoided.*]

P–20. Sure, they're afraid of me. When I came here, they took tests. What did they prove?

N–21. That you're not well and need psychiatric help. [*The nurse is attempting to convince the patient that he is sick.*]

P–22. I think Dr. _____ is one of those devils. Mr. _____ has sparkle of the devil in his eyes. The perversion that is going on is disgusting me. They're afraid of me.

N–23. Why do you think they are? [*Requesting an explanation. Trying to find out why he thinks others are afraid of him.*]

P–24. I'm big.

N–25. You're not that big. [*Challenging. The patient may need to think that the "devils" or "perverted ones" are afraid, to keep them away from him. The nurse should determine what he is afraid of—what he has to be powerful for.*]

P–26. Those four devils are threatening weaker ones to kill me and get judgment. _____ is the original devil.

N–27. Lucifer. [*Verbalizing the implied. This seems, however, to indicate that the nurse agrees.*]

P–28. Yes. What time is it now?

N–29. 10:45. [*Giving information.*]

P–30. Mass is being said now for the dead. (Looking to the sun.)

N–31. What if nothing happens? [*Challenging.*]

P–32. Something is going to happen. It almost happened yesterday. In the mess hall last evening—no, at lunchtime—there was a knife play between A. and B. A. was next to me. B. was across the table. A. was on my side—yes, supper last night. Aides ——, ——, and —— luckily spotted knife, and anything can happen in a knife fight. I felt they may have drained my blood. That's why I asked to have it taken medically. That x-ray man is also the devil. If I'm going to die, I don't want to die rough. I was rushed into hospital protection.

N–33. From whom? [*Seeking clarification. The patient is expressing fear of being assaulted.*]

P–34. Those four devils. I can get my kid, and he can identify him as being on my street in ——. All this started when I was in Kansas City.

N–35. Why? [*Requesting an explanation. This comment is inappropriate. It is more important to find out what happened before the nurse tries to understand why.*]

P–36. Because time is near. I have nothing to worry about because the good Lord is watching over me.

N–37. I must leave you now. I'll be seeing you again soon. [*This is an abrupt closing. The nurse should attempt to summarize what has transpired and be more specific as to when he will return.*]

P–38. Adios.

Despite the many shortcomings, the patient seems to have accepted the nurse as someone in whom to confide. There is progress. He is trying to communicate with another human being—the nurse.

The nurse must see that the patient continues to communicate. When an idea is not understood, it must be clarified. The patient should not be permitted to go ahead without clarifying each step. The amount of ground covered is not the important consideration. It is better to get one point mutually understood than to discuss several topics meaninglessly. The nurse should explore the personal references—how this and that apply to the patient and to his life.

The patient may feel the need to be a powerful person to prevent something from happening. The nurse must keep this idea in mind and explore it when the opportunity presents itself.

It is also important to indicate to the patient that he can be liked for himself. Communicating to him that he does not need to be perfect or invincible to succeed in life is to be considered. The nurse should help him see his accomplishments—his job, his family. The relationship should indicate to the patient that he is liked, that his difficulties are not insurmountable, and that help is available.

Twelfth Day

N–1. Good morning, Al. How's everything? [*Giving recognition and an opening.*]

P–2. Good morning, Mr. L.

N–3. What would you care to discuss today? [*The nurse's broad opening gives the patient an opportunity to take the initiative.*]

P–4. It's up to you. (Appearing annoyed.)

N–5. Has Dr. ____ given you a treatment? [*The nurse has taken the initiative and is seeking information. It would have been preferable to find out why the patient appeared annoyed.*]

P–6. I've been getting it on Monday and Wednesday.

N–7. Is there anything you'd particularly like to discuss about treatments? [*Asking the patient for his reaction to the topic introduced.*]

P–8. I just black out, and I'm the same then as when I went to sleep. Is it supposed to make me forget?

P–9. No. It's supposed to help relieve some of one's anxiety and tensions. [*Giving information about the treatment. The nurse might add, "The forgetting, if it occurs, will only be temporary."*]

P–10. I saw those other guys carrying on—moaning and groaning.

N–11. How does it feel? [*Encouraging description of perceptions. Better worded, "What feelings do you have?"*]

P–12. No feelings whatsoever. Blacking out and waking up.

N–13. Do you still see people the same way? [*The nurse is testing to see if the patient continues to be delusional. The response is as vague as the nurse's question. The patient's reply is appropriate if he feels that he sees people the same way he always has. Consequently, the nurse has not learned anything from this exchange.*]

P–14. Yes. Still the same. (Silence.)

N–15. Would you like to discuss your job? What they thought of your work and such? [*Introducing a new topic. Apparently the patient has lost interest in what the nurse has brought up.*]

P–16. They have no complaints. I'm still top man.

N–17. What type of work do they do? [*Seeking information. The nurse continues to use the vague "they."*]

P–18. They do all big jobs—hospitals and schools.

N–19. How did you and your boss get along? [*Asking the patient to evaluate his relationship with his boss.*]

P–20. Okay. He expected you to work. I gave an honest day's work and no more.

N–21. Did anything happen that would lead you to believe that you were not doing your share? [*Exploring. The nurse has taken a clue and is examining what has been said. This is appropriate.*]

P–22. He insinuated I could do more.

N–23. How did he do that? [*Seeking clarification.*]

P–24. With his mouth. He'd say I thought you'd have that done today.

N–25. Did this annoy you? [*The nurse is trying to have the patient describe his feelings.*]

P–26. Yes. I told him not to worry about it.

N–27. Did he say these things in front of other people? [*The nurse continues to seek further description of the situation.*]

P–28. No. He took me aside. He'd gotten rapped if he didn't. He changed his name to B. He had some foreign name. I wouldn't change my name for all the money in the world. There's a woman in charge. She's the boss. She changed her name after her husband died. She's better than her brother. They're Christians. Catholics.

N–29. How does your boss get along in the shop? [*Directing the conversation back to the subject of his boss.*]

P–30. He creates tensions in the shop. He thinks he knows the business, but he doesn't.

N–31. Do you find it hard to work under such tension? [*Verbalizing the implied. Exploring the patient's feelings in the work situation.*]

P–32. Yes, but I still gave a good day's work.

N–33. I've got to leave you now, Al. I'll be seeing you.

P–34. So long, Mr. L.

The nurse has followed through on a topic and was able to uncover a troublesome relationship of the patient's. This discovery might explain why he needs to build up the delusion that he is perfect and blameless. It is important to determine how others felt about this man. The nurse should also explore and examine the relationship the patient had with his co-workers and with those who worked under his supervision.

Thirteenth Day

N–1. Good morning, Al. How are you doing? [*Giving recognition. Broad opening comment. "How are you doing?" is a stereotyped question. It receives a stereotyped answer.*]

P–2. Fine.

N–3. I guess you must have wondered what happened to me, as I haven't spent much time with you. [*The nurse should periodically remind the patient of the purpose of the time being spent with him.*]

P–4. No. You must have been busy. You know I'm losing a lot of money staying here. About a $150 a week take home. That ain't hay.

N–5. I know you must be concerned about this, Al, but you must also think about your personal health. [*Advising. Accepting the patient's feeling of concern but suggesting that his health is more important. However, the nurse should be alert to the fact that the patient may take "health" to mean physical well-being. If such is the case, the two participants are talking about different subjects.*]

P–6. I feel fine.

N–7. Well, you certainly look fine. [*Agreeing. The patient may assume that the nurse is saying that he is well. It is better to indicate progress, when warranted, by saying, "You appear more relaxed" rather than indicating that his present condition is "good."*]

P–8. I got popped in the jaw this morning.

N–9. By whom? [*Exploring.*]

P–10. A. Going into the mess hall, B. was pushing my wheelchair, and he accidentally ran over A.'s feet, and he hauls off and slugs me. The aides stopped me from retaliating. All I wanted was one punch, but that's how it goes.

N–11. You don't seem too upset over it now, so I guess all is forgiven? [*Making an observation. The nurse is tentatively suggesting an explanation for his not seeming upset.*]

P–12. Yeah.

N–13. Well, that's a good sign, Al. I'm glad to see you feel that way. [*The nurse is voicing his approval. This can be overdone, resulting in the patient's feeling that too much is expected of him—that the nurse will be disapproving if he loses control in the future. The nurse could have led up to a discussion of what kind of things upset him and how he usually expresses his anger.*]

P–14. Shows Al S.'s getting on the ball. How many more treatments do I have to have, or don't you know?

N–15. Well, a series is usually 20 treatments, but it depends on how well the patient does during the course of treatment. If there is a great improvement, they won't give an entire series. So you see, it's an individual thing. [*Giving information. Again the use of "they" is vague when the nurse might very well have said that it is the doctor's decision.*]

P–16. Well, I've had about eight, and I'm feeling fine.

N–17. Is there anything else that makes you feel that Al S. is on the ball? [*The patient is given an opportunity to evaluate his progress as he sees it.*]

P–18. Yes. We need ashtrays around here.

N–19. What else has happened that makes you say that you're getting back on the ball? [*Encouraging description of perceptions.*]

P–20. Christmas is coming, and I want to go home to my kids and wife. I don't want to spend the holidays here, that's for certain. My attitude has changed. Some of these fellows are way out. I humor them along. I don't get into conversation with them.

N–21. How are they way out? [*Seeking clarification. Better worded, "In what way . . . ?"*]

P–22. The way they talk to me.

N–23. How is that? [*Asking the patient to be specific.*]

P–24. They don't talk sensible.

N–25. How was your attitude before? [*Encouraging comparison. "What was . . . ?"*]

P–26. Well, I was going to lead them on a major break out of the hospital, which wouldn't have been hard to do.

N–27. Do you think they would have followed? [*Exploring.*]

P–28. Sure, they would have. I was way out too though.

N–29. How about describing to me how "way out" you were, if you can? [*The nurse is encouraging self-evaluation and description.*]

P–30. I felt I was being persecuted.

N–31. By whom? [*Exploring source.*]

P–32. By the doctors, especially when they restrained me with the sheet and packs.

N–33. Do you realize why it had to be done? It's only to protect you, the property, and other people and not for punitive measures. [*Testing and defending. It would have been better to have accepted the patient's feeling by saying something such as "I guess it did seem unfair," then noting that it was for his own protection. "I can see what you might have felt" would also have been an appropriate response. Otherwise, it may seem that the nurse is siding with those who seem to be persecuting him.*]

P–34. I don't feel that way now, though. I don't have any use for Dr. _____. Have you ever made rounds with him?

N–35. I've made rounds with him, but have not noticed anything unusual about him. [*The nurse mentions his experience without disagreeing with the patient.*]

P–36. You know something else that made me feel persecuted was the way you operate here. If they would have taken me and showed me how they operate here, it would have been easier because you wouldn't have had the trouble with me you did. I was way out, and I asked them to do away with me.

N–37. This indicates you needed help. When did this feeling of wanting to do away with yourself start? [*The nurse introduces a related topic. Placing event in time.*]

P–38. I can't remember back that far. (Thinking.)

N–39. It wasn't too long ago. [*The nurse is implying that he should remember.*]

P–40. No, I know.

N–41. What do you think made you seek help here? [*Testing insight.*]

P–42. I can't remember. Maybe it was too much drinking.

N–43. Was it heavier than usual? [*Encouraging comparison.*]

P–44. No.

N–45. Then why do you think that drinking started to get you? [*Requesting an explanation.*]

P–46. Accumulation. I had stopped before I came in. When I got back from Kansas City, I stopped.

N–47. Why? [*Requesting an explanation.*]

P–48. I had no desire.

N–49. Were you frightened about anything that would make you stop? [*The nurse is suggesting a possible explanation.*]

P–50. You mean the lightning or the music. No, I had just lost the desire. That's when I felt they were after me.

N–51. Who? [*Seeking clarification.*]

P–52. Well, when I was in Kansas City I went out looking for women and dope—just to try it. I met some bad boys (smiling) at a gin mill. I was throwing money around like water, and I think I made a contact for some dope which I never did get. I thought they were going to get me.

N–53. What do you mean, "bad boys"? [*Seeking clarification. The nurse's question is appropriate. Since "What do you mean" tends to be intimidating, however, the nurse could ask, "What are you referring to when you say 'bad boys'?"*]

P–54. They were pushers who had guns. The women were all in on it, and you could see for yourself. It was real disgusting, and I couldn't touch any of them. When I got back, I went to the police to report it. I then went to ____ Hospital to rest up.

N–55. Did you start drinking when you were home? [*Exploring. It might have been of more value for the nurse to explore further what the patient told the police and their reaction, and other events that led to his admission. The connection is not clear.*]

P–56. No.

N–57. What happened at this public party you went to just before you came here? [*Introducing a related event.*]

P–58. It was my son's fire department's picnic, and there was a lot of dancing and stuff going on. I didn't care for it too much, and I told them I wanted to go home.

N–59. I thought you became unconscious. [*The nurse has introduced information that has not been gained from this relationship but rather from his clinical chart. It is better not to introduce this information. If the patient feels that what was told to a physician in confidence is known by others, or that information given by his family is common knowledge, he has a right to become annoyed.*]

P–60. I made believe I passed out. I wanted to go home and I did. The next day I came here on my own.

N–61. Did you have any feelings about desiring dope and women while you were in Kansas City? [*The patient is being asked to describe his feelings. Better worded, "What were your feelings about . . . ?"*]

P–62. This is a normal feeling, but those poor women stuffed with dope disgusted me.

N–63. You felt that the men in the gin mill were following you on your way to work. [*The nurse again refers to information not gained from the relationship.*]

P–64. Yes. I used to go the same way to work all the time. This day I noticed these sports cars following me; so I decided to go another way, which I did, and they kept on coming. (Becoming very firm and convinced.) No one can tell me that they were not following me.

N–65. Al, I'd like to explain something to you about similar circumstances that have happened to me and a lot of other people, I'm sure. I've driven along and happened to see cars in my rear-view mirror that appeared to be following me. This is apparently an imaginary thing. I'd stop or turn, and a car would follow, and it would appear to be following. However, it would always prove to be imaginary. [*The nurse is attempting to present reality by describing his own experiences.*]

P–66. (Period of thought.) I guess you're right. [*An element of doubt was introduced as to the reality of the patient's experience. It was accepted and acknowledged.*]

N–67. I'm sure I am, Al. It just seemed this way to you. I must go now. [*The nurse is giving the impression of being infallible. What started out as presenting reality has turned into an attempt to convince the patient.*]

The nurse-patient relationship is developing. The nurse is keeping the patient focused on a particular area for considerable lengths of time. The patient is being followed up on what he says, and the nurse is gaining some real understanding of how things appear to him. The nurse seems to be concentrating on the patient, and he is responding to the interest shown.

Fourteenth Day

N–1. Buenos tardes, amigo. That's Spanish for "Good afternoon, friend."

P–2. (Laughing.) What the hell are you doing here today?

N–3. Well, it happens to the best of us here where we're called to duty on Sunday. Not as often as other people, but every now and then. Once in about eight weeks. [*The nurse gives information. His reference to "the best of us" might have been better omitted.*]

P–4. That's not bad.

N–5. No. This job is something like yours. Work half a day and rest the rest. [*The nurse broadens the topic to include the patient's job. However, the patient expressed concern when he spoke of being questioned by his boss about how fast he could do a job. The nurse should save his humor for a different topic.*]

P–6. (He laughed and appeared in good spirits.)

N–7. Do you ever play cards with the other patients? [*Introducing an unrelated topic. The nurse is exploring his relationship with other patients.*]

P–8. No, I wasn't much for cards even in the service.

N–9. Where did you serve? [*Exploring. The patient has offered the nurse a lead, and the nurse responds appropriately.*]

P–10. Hawaii, Canton, Okinawa. I was about a year in Hawaii. I didn't want to be called a fairy, so I asked for active duty. I got it all right. I was in the invasion of Okinawa.

N–11. What day? [*Exploring. The nurse should have been concerned* *with the homosexual connotation. Was it merely because the patient had an easy assignment that he was concerned?*]

P–12. D plus four.

N–13. What did you do? [*Encouraging description.*]

P–14. We shuttled supplies to the front lines. When I asked for active duty, I told the commanding officer he had a chicken outfit and everything else. So he fixed me up. (Smiling.) I was outspoken.

N–15. When did you change? [*Seeking comparison. This comment has the effect of changing the subject. The patient's service experiences certainly warrant further exploration when he brings the topic up again.*]

P–16. When I started earning a living. I was a plumber's helper, and I worked my tail off. You don't say much under those conditions. I learned my trade for five years. This was after I got out of the service. I had two brothers and a father and mother to support.

N–17. You contributed quite a bit to their economy? [*Restating what the patient has implied.*]

P–18. When I was in the Army and Merchant Marine, I sent home an allotment check.

N–19. Was your father working? [*Seeking information.*]

P–20. No. He was a heavy drinker, but he was sickly. He had ulcers.

N–21. From what? [*Testing. Exploring the patient's knowledge of the problems associated with the excessive use of alcohol.*]

P–22. Drinking. My uncle was the same way. It's funny we should be talking about my father because just last visiting day my wife came and said "Al S., you look just like your father!" She took care of him when he had a stroke. We bathed him and did everything else. They wouldn't accept him in any hospital because the doctor said why prolong the inevitable. He didn't believe we should hospitalize him. We gave him Demerol and kept him doped up. That's all there was to that. He died three months after his stroke.

N–23. Where did he live? [*Seeking information.*]

P–24. He lived with me.

N–25. What did he do around the house? [*Seeking information. It would have been of more value for the nurse to learn of the patient's feelings toward his father and the kind of relationship they had.*]

P–26. He was very handy. Did odd jobs. Drank. Every penny he got went to drink. (It was announced that the patient had a visitor.) Why don't you come down and meet her?

N–27. All right. I'll be right there. [*The patient's invitation indicates that the nurse's relationship with him has importance for him.*]

It is obvious that the nurse and the patient are gaining something from this relationship. The patient has not spoken about the devils and being Jesus for some time. It may be that he no longer needs to be perfect and infallible.

There are many areas of the patient's life that are worth exploring, but only when he brings them up: for example, the patient's relationship with significant people in his childhood (mother, father, siblings), his service experience (authority, his buddies), his job (co-workers, boss, those under him), and his marriage (wife, children). It can be said that the nurse at this point has developed a nurse-patient relationship that has therapeutic potential.

Fifteenth Day

N–1. Hello, Al. How's everything? [*Given recognition. Broad opening comment.*]

P–2. Did you hear? I get grounds pass with my wife. How about that?

N–3. You know how I feel. I think it's terrific, and it sure shows that you've come a long way. I'm really thrilled by your success. When was this all decided? [*Giving approval. It might have been better for the nurse to have said, "You certainly seem happy about it" or something of this sort. It is difficult, and understandably so, not to pat the patient on the back. However, approval can sometimes backfire. The relationship is improved when all is going well. But if the patient does again become more disturbed, he will expect the nurse's disapproval.*]

P–4. Friday! They had staff and decided I was a good boy, and they were going to leave it in Dr. S.'s hands. When I went in for shock this morning, I asked him about going on the grounds pass with my wife, and he said yes, it was approved.

N–5. That wasn't all the staff decided, was it? [*Testing. The nurse seems to imply that he already knows of the staff's decision. If he does, he could have said, "They decided more than that at staff, I hear." If he does not, the nurse could have said, "Did the doctors decide anything else?"*]

P–6. They removed me from maximum supervision status and transferred me to another unit.

N–7. To what can we attribute your success and progress? [*The nurse is asking the patient to identify the source of his progress. It would have been more suitable to ask what he attributes his progress to, rather than suggest "we."*]

P–8. Prayers to the Lord. (Removing prayer book from pocket.) I got this from Father. . . . (Pause. Appearing annoyed.) Damn that shock; I can't remember.

N–9. Father M. [*Giving information.*]

P–10. Yes. Father M. I read the morning and night prayers, and it sure has helped. My wife is very pleased and happy with me.

N–11. So am I, Al. It's very encouraging to all of us to see someone like yourself improve as you have. [*Giving approval. The nurse can give recognition to the patient's progress by noting how he seems "more relaxed," "more comfortable," "under less tension," etc. Otherwise, it implies to the patient approval for good behavior and disappointment with "sick" behavior. To say "someone like yourself" implies that he is very much different from others. It is, therefore, better omitted.*]

P–12. Thank you. Dr. K. asked me if I was mad at H. I said, "No, I'm not mad at him. I can see him being angry because I went over his foot. He's mentally ill." (Silence.) How are you?

N–13. Well, except for a persistent sinus headache, I can't complain. [*Allowing conversation to focus on the nurse. The nurse should have considered the patient's question as being merely an attempt to break the silence. He should be told that the time is to be used to discuss his problems not the nurse's.*]

P–14. I once had a sinus headache, but I never had it come back.

N–15. When was this? [*Placing the event in time.*]

P–16. Some time back; I can't remember. You don't happen to pass my school?

N–17. Yes, as a matter of fact, I saw three men standing about talking last Sunday. [*Giving information. The patient is expressing interest in his work. This would have been a good time for the nurse to see what his feelings were about it.*]

P–18. The roughing must be done by now, and they should be starting on the finishings. That's the gravy train. What's remotivation—for employees?

N–19. (Smiling.) Al, do you think our employees need motivating?

P–20. (Laughing.) Some do.

N–21. It's a program that the aides are trained in and some nurses. They gather a group of patients together and determine what the chief interest of the group is. Then after some research and preparation, they hold a group discussion. It's quite interesting and takes a lot of effort on the part of the personnel. We find the patients very interested and anxious to attend. Maybe you can ask Mr. G. to attend some. [*Giving information. The program is well described and offers the patient an opportunity to be included. The presentation of material in an enthusiastic manner will help him decide how to occupy his time in the hospital.*]

P–22. I'll do that. You know this is the first Christmas party I'll be missing. It's held for the officers of the union, and this would have been the first year for me. But I guess it's more important that I be home with my family. (Pause.) You know when that patient that burned himself came here, they held a shakedown that was a shakedown. They got a lighter from me. I only had it to save the aides some time.

N–23. You can understand why we don't permit the patients to have matches here. [*Indicating that he does not feel the patient requires an explanation.*] How did you get a lighter? [*Exploring.*]

P–24. My brother gave it to me. Mrs. D. told me she has it locked up and will give it to me to return home.

N–25. Does your wife know about your good fortune? [*The nurse introduces a topic related to what has been discussed.*]

P–26. No. Some surprise! I've been surprising her all my life—coming here was a surprise and a shock. I thought it was for an examination, not to be kept here.

N–27. You don't object too much to staying here now? [*The nurse should avoid making positive statements like this. It would have been better to have replied, "You don't seem to object . . ." or something of this nature. Another suggestion is that the nurse might acknowledge that this hospitalization must have been quite a shock to him. In addition, such comments as "I would imagine it'd be quite disturbing" or "I guess it must have made you angry" would have given the patient an opportunity to verbalize his feelings.*]

P–28. No, it won't be too much longer. The way things are going, it seems that things are really moving. You have no idea what this place was like over the week end. Everyone screaming for paraldehyde. D. over there moaning. Some week end! This was a real madhouse. That guy P. was loaded with paraldehyde. He must have been on some toot. Do you know what I'm going to do when I get out?

N–29. No, what? [*Giving a general lead.*]

P–30. I'm going to take my wife on a trip. No, first I'm going to take a week's rest. Then I'm going to Florida.

N–31. Have you ever been there? [*Seeking information. Giving the patient a chance to bring up his past experiences.*]

P–32. Yes, in the Merchant Marine.

N–33. How old were you? [*Exploring. The nurse is placing the event in time.*]

P–34. I was 16. I ran away from home.

N–35. Why? [*Requesting an explanation. "Tell me about this," the nurse might have said.*]

P–36. Well, I got in some trouble in school.

N–37. What kind? [*Exploring.*]

P–38. I was in the hospital with an appendectomy, and on my first day back to school a guy kicked me in the stomach. I beat the hell out of him and knocked his eye out. I was told to go home and bring my father. I took off. My father'd knock my tail off. I stayed in the city.

N–39. Where? [*Seeking more specific details. The nurse might have explored this event further. This incident must have been quite traumatic to the patient. From here the nurse could have gone into his relationships with the boys and girls in school. Also, more could have been learned of the patient's relationship with his father by stating something similar to "I guess your father wouldn't have understood." The patient needs the nurse to help him verbalize the feelings he had toward the boy and toward his own father.*]

P–40. Downtown.

N–41. How'd you live? [*Exploring.*]

P–42. I held odd jobs. When the war broke out, I tried to join the Navy, but they turned me down. So I enlisted in the Merchant Marine.

N–43. Since you felt the way you did toward your father, why did you send your money home? [*Requesting an explanation. The nurse, in saying "since you felt so about your father," is being very vague. The patient has not really expressed his feeling about his father. If the patient was fearful of him, it would have been well to find out if the feeling was of long standing.*]

P–44. He had small kids to care for, but I went home after my tour in the Merchant Marine. He drank most of it up anyway, but the kids ate first. I then went to work in ____'s, and this was some comedown. Twenty-five dollars a week. They drafted me soon after.

N–45. Then you drove the ferry in Hawaii. [*Recalling what occurred next from previous conversations.*]

P–46. Yes. What a racket!

N–47. How did your buddies feel about your racket? [*The nurse is asking the patient to evaluate the situation and his relationships at the time.*]

P–48. They thought I was crazy to ask for action.

N–49. Why did you? [*Requesting an explanation.*]

P–50. I was tired of sitting around doing nothing. So I did.

N–51. Well, Al, I admire your spirit. I must be leaving now. I'm very satisfied with the good news. Almost as much as you are. I'll see you soon. [*Giving approval.*]

N–52. So long, ____.

The patient seems to feel that he is well. The nurse's approval may make him feel that he agrees. Hence, the patient may feel that he is not supposed to have any problems. The nurse can acknowledge any apparent improvement by noting specific ways in which his behavior is different from what it was previously.

The nurse should consider spending the remaining time of this relationship in exploring further the problems the patient still has. The patient is going back, eventually, to the environment and problems that made him sick. The relationship has not given the nurse any information concerning these areas.

When the opportunities present themselves, it would be helpful for the nurse to have the patient discuss such matters as the kinds of people with whom he feels uncomfortable, the kinds of situations or people that make him feel inadequate or inferior, what things make him feel angry, what he does when he gets angry, what he expects from himself—his goals, etc.—and why he needed to drink excessively.

When the patient speaks of going home and being well, the nurse might mention that his illness was not something strange and mysterious that came upon him from nowhere and now has left or is leaving him, but that such illnesses develop out of difficult and unhappy relationships with people, and that by his discussing what some of these problems were, he can better understand how they made him so anxious that he had to become sick, and that such understanding will make illness less likely to occur again.

The patient appears to have approached the time when he is in good enough contact to work with the nurse on understanding his problems better through this nurse-patient relationship.

Sixteenth Day

N–1. Hi, Al. How are things? [*Giving recognition and opening comment.*]

P–2. Just fine.

N–3. How was your week end? [*Seeking information. The nurse has taken the initiative. The nurse can break the ice with a few opening comments but should note when the opening comments are over. The nurse appears to drift aimlessly into conversation, exploring whenever a topic strikes him as being of importance. It gives the patient no idea of his reasons for such questioning and may put him on the defensive or at least make him uneasy. The nurse never explains what he is doing or why he is doing it. It would be more advantageous for the nurse to tell the patient that he spends time with him so that together they can explore *the problems he has had with people so that he can better understand himself. The patient can be told that this may help him understand his illness and also help him to be less likely to be sick again. Otherwise, it may just seem like meaningless prying on the part of the nurse, which the patient tolerates because he may happen to like the nurse in spite of it.*]

P–4. My wife and children were here, and they pushed me to the canteen. My brother, Jimmy, was here also.

N–5. Which one is Jimmy? [*Seeking clarification.*]

P–6. He's third youngest. (He mentioned his brothers' names including one who was killed in another state.)

N–7. H. was the one who was killed in Virginia, wasn't he? [*Focusing on a particular brother.*]

P–8. Yes.

N–9. What happened? [*Exploring. Encouraging description but of a topic chosen by the nurse.*]

P–10. From what I was told by his buddy, there were two guys sitting in this barroom. They had offered this girl a drink, and she refused. My brother and his buddy were on their way back to camp from a movie when my brother wanted to stop for a beer. He went into the place where the two guys were, and when the woman refused them, he offered to buy one for her. She refused but said she would take a drink from his. One of the two guys asked the other if he should give it to him now, and the other said "Yeah." So they shot him in the abdomen.

N–11. Were you and your brother attached? [*The nurse is exploring the depth of the relationship.*]

P–12. Very much so.

N–13. How did this make you feel? [*Asking the patient to evaluate his feelings. "What were your feelings?"*]

P–14. Bad.

N–15. Can you describe this bad feeling? [*Encouraging description. Seeking clarification. The nurse is appropriately asking the patient to try to put feelings into the word "bad."*]

P–16. I felt very bad. All wrought up. I wanted to go to Virginia and get locked up and get this guy. But everyone—my wife, brothers, father—convinced me I should stay home. They told me it was God's will, and that everything would be taken care of. That's pretty good reasoning, but when I look at the missal here—that's a coincidence because that's Bobby's birthday. (Patient showed set of numbers found in the Catholic missal.)

N–17. I don't know what it means, but it doesn't have any bearing on your brother's death. [*The nurse is attempting to give information. How-*

ever, he does not appear to be on very firm ground in view of his lack of information about the subject mentioned. It would have been better to reply, "It would seem very unlikely that it has any bearing on. . . ." The nurse should not feel that he has or must have all the answers. When such situations do arise, the nurse can readily admit his lack of knowledge but assure the patient that efforts will be made to obtain the information requested.]

P–18. I'll have to ask the priest what it means.

N–19. How long afterward did you stay angry? [*The nurse has directed the patient back to the subject under discussion.*]

P–20. About a year. I was very angry.

N–21. Can you describe this anger? [*Encouraging description. Exploring. Feelings, particularly of such magnitude, are always worth further exploration. The nurse can rarely go wrong or waste time by looking into them more deeply and getting the patient to verbalize what he feels.*]

P–22. I could have torn him apart.

N–23. What happened to the man? [*Seeking information.*]

P–24. He got 20 years in. . . . What's the capitol?

N–25. I can't remember either. [*The nurse admits his own lack of information.*]

P–26. Jesus, I was stationed down there. (Silence.) Richmond, that's it!

N–27. Has any other situation made you as angry as this? [*Encouraging comparison. This was a very timely query. The nurse focused on the patient's anger throughout this discussion. This is admittedly an area of difficulty for the patient.*]

P–28. No. The only other incident that made me as angry was moving me from Ward _____ to this ward. They should have sent me to a better ward like _____ or _____. I can't understand why they made the move. You can ask Mr. _____. He said I was all right.

N–29. How were you angry? [*Exploring. Encouraging description. Better worded, "In what way. . . ?" or "Tell me about your anger."*]

P–30. I kept myself cool until I saw Dr. _____ and asked for privileges. Everything built up all at once, and then they denied my request to drain my blood, and you know what happened. I didn't hurt or want to hurt anybody. I could have, but I was in a property-destroying mood. You can ask Mr. _____. My ideas now is to get straightened out, leave here, and go back to my wife and family and my job.

N–31. What else has happened to you that has raised your anger? [*The nurse continues to focus on the topic of anger, but it would also* *have been worthwhile pursuing his comment, "Everything built up all at once. . . ."*]

P–32. I used to visit this one gin mill regularly. For about two and a half years.

N–33. What happened? [*Exploring. Encouraging description.*]

P–34. Well, this ex-German-U-boat commander was mouthing off and knocking the United States, the Army, Marines, me—and I wouldn't stand for it. He was a big powerful S.O.B. I asked him outside, and he and I went round and round. This was about four years ago. He said enough to get you irritated, especially if you're half bagged.

N–35. Were you? [*Seeking information.*]

P–36. Yes.

N–37. Any other time? [*Exploring.*]

P–38. Yes, I got angry at a mess sergeant once when he refused to give me seconds. We had returned from a 15-mile hike, and I was hungry. He refused, so we stepped outside and had it out. It was broken up by a second lieutenant, and I was confined to quarters. I went over the hill though, and when I got back, I got company punishment. I had to scrub down the duckwalk for two weeks.

N–39. What happened to the mess sergeant? [*Seeking information. Exploring.*]

P–40. Nothing. I also had a fight in the Merchant Marine with a cook over food.

N–41. Did you win that fight? [*Seeking information. Exploring.*]

P–42. Yes.

N–43. Have you ever lost? [*Seeking information. The nurse is getting away from the central issue. It is not the patient's strength or his courage that is important. What the nurse should be interesed in discovering is the kind of things that make him angry. So far the patient has indicated that anything that makes him feel others are considering him inferior or less worthwhile than other people makes him angry. This would have been an opportune time to ask the patient directly if there are any similarities, any common element in these situations in which he became angry.*]

P–44. No. Once when I was 12, I picked on a guy who was a good fighter, and he gave me a lesson.

N–45. Was it easy to take? [*Asking the patient to evaluate the situation. Perhaps better worded, "What were your feelings about this?"*]

P–46. It wasn't easy, but I took it.

N–47. That fight you had in school—were you angry at that boy? [*Exploring the patient's anger further.*]

P–48. I sure was.

N–49. Why didn't you go home to your father? Didn't you think you were right? [*Requesting an explanation. The nurse is changing the topic of conversation somewhat.*]

P–50. I was afraid he'd kick the ____ out of me.

N–51. Had he before? [*Exploring. Seeking information.*]

P–52. Sure.

N–53. How did you feel about him? [*The nurse is asking the patient to evaluate his feelings toward his father. It would be useful for the nurse to know the kinds of things his father beat him for. Better worded, "What were your feelings. . . ?"*]

P–54. I loved him. He wasn't bad. He was better drunk than sober. My brother lost his toes because he got into trouble and was afraid to go home one winter. He spent a year in the hospital. My father was strict. He didn't pull punches.

N–55. Would you consider him fair? [*Seeking further evaluation, however, the nurse is asking the kinds of questions that tend to produce stereotyped answers. It would be worthwhile to explore further the patient's being "afraid" of his father. What did his father expect from him? Why was he afraid? What did he expect might happen? Did he feel he had to be perfect? In what ways did he fall short?*]

P–56. Yes, he was fair.

N–57. Are you like him? [*Encouraging comparison.*]

P–58. No, I'm myself.

N–59. How do you differ? [*The patient's previous comment implies that he accepts his own identity. The nurse explores further by encouraging comparison. Better worded, "In what way . . . ?"*]

P–60. I stick more to a job. He got paid and drank his check away. That's one thing I never did.

N–61. How did you get money to drink? [*Probing. The nurse is changing the topic of conversation.*]

P–62. Tips.

N–63. What we men call mad money? [*The nurse is indicating that he follows.*]

P–64. I made up my mind I'm going to stop drinking. I haven't had any since I came back from Kansas City.

N–65. That's a good start, Al. I'm afraid I must leave you now. It's been a pleasure as usual. [*Giving approval.*]

The nurse should plan to close each meeting with a summary rather than close abruptly every time. The nurse should take stock with the patient of what has transpired. Nurse and patient should explore together what was discussed—sum it up—and see whether they both have the same impressions and plan where to go from there.

Seventeenth Day

(The patient was selecting a book from the library cart when the nurse entered the ward.)

N–1. Take your time, Al. [*The nurse is allowing the patient to take the initiative in approaching him when he is ready.*]

P–2. Look what that _____ did to my missal. (Many names of the patient's family were written through it.)

N–3. How did he get to know all the names of your family? [*Seeking clarification.*]

P–4. I guess through some small talk.

N–5. Do you do much reading? [*Exploring the patient's interests. It is better not to ask questions that can be answered "Yes" or "no." Not much information is obtained, and the nurse ends up having to ask question after question.*]

P–6. Yes.

N–7. Anything in particular? [*Exploring further.*]

P–8. I like historical novels.

N–9. Can you remember any names? [*The nurse seems to be pressing.*]

P–10. Offhand, no. (Pause.) I've read Genghis Khan, the Crusades. If I could take you home, I'd show you. (The ward nurse entered and gave the patient his medication.) You know when they were giving me 300 mg four times a day, it was too much because I was getting jumpy.

N–11. Do you mean listless? [*Seeking clarification. The nurse is trying to determine whether the patient is using the right word to describe the effect of the drug.*]

P–12. No, jumpy. So I made believe I took it. Finally I told them, and they gave me the liquid. Now it's down to 300 mg a day.

N–13. Would you take it at home if the doctors feel it's necessary? [*Testing.*]

P–14. If they give it to me and feel it's necessary, sure I will. I want to get out of here. But before I go, I want to have both feet on the ground. [*The patient's reply is interesting. The nurse might have followed it up by asking something like, "Your present feelings are not comfortable ones?" or "In what ways would you like to feel differently than you do now?"*]

N–15. We'll try to get both feet on the ground, but you must remember that when you leave, you're going to return to work, your home, and just about everything you left. You also will be exposed to many of the problems and joys you had before, and you must be ready to expect this. [*Reassuring. The patient is informed that he will receive some vague form of assistance; then the nurse points out possible pitfalls, in a vague way. Consequently, there is no real follow-up. The nurse says there will be problems; the patient says, "I know." The nurse might have been more direct and asked, "What do you think will be your biggest problem when you get home?"*]

P–16. I know this, and if I feel I need help, I'll be back.

N–17. That's very wise, Al, and certainly shows good sense on your part. [*Giving approval. The nurse implies that the patient had not had "good sense" previously. It might have been better to explore further how he will recognize the need for help in the future.*]

P–18. I handled them before. I can do it again.

N–19. Have you had any further thoughts about what you're going to do when you leave? [*Encouraging the formulation of a plan for the future.*]

P–20. I'm going home for a week and then back to work.

N–21. What happened to the trip to Florida with your wife? [*Exploring. The patient seems to feel less of a need now for a period of recuperation before returning to his job.*]

P–22. If she wants to go, I'll take her. You know my job may not want me back.

N–23. Why? [*Requesting an explanation. The patient has expressed his real worry. The nurse asks for his reasoning.*]

P–24. Because they know I'm an inmate at _____. They have some poor ideas about you when you're hospitalized.

N–25. It's too bad they can't consider this like having an appendectomy or an attack of diabetes. Both call for one to be hospitalized and sometimes care for the rest of one's life. [*The patient may be projecting his own sense of shame. The nurse should attempt to find out whether this is realistic or not. Has the patient seen anyone or had any word that would support his doubts?*]

P–26. When I first came in here, they called home a lot of times looking for me. I guess they got a guy from the shop to take my place. I had the job well advanced so that anyone taking my place would just have to take it easy.

N–27. Do you have any doubts about getting a job again? [*Asking the patient to evaluate his ability to get work. The patient says he can, but he does seem concerned. The patient does not want just his job back,* *rather, the patient does not want to lose status, to be rejected by his boss and other people. His concern seems to be about more than earning a living. The nurse might have explored this further by asking something like, "Then what is it that really bothers you?" or "You don't want to lose this job, do you? What would losing it mean to you?"*]

P–28. No. If the company I worked for doesn't take me back, I can always get work. I'm on the executive board, so I should be able to find something. They offered me a pension when I was on Ward ____, but I didn't apply. Not as long as I feel I can work. I told them what they can do with it. I can support my family myself.

N–29. I'm sure you'll be able to do all right for yourself, Al. It's a good thing to know that you have the interest of the government if you are not able to get work. So you know who you can go to if such is the case. I feel that you should find suitable employment when you leave. [*Reassuring. The nurse says that he is sure the patient can get work and then introduces an element of doubt by telling him that if he cannot, the government will take care of him. The nurse should not give reassurance that has no foundation in fact.*]

Eighteenth Day

N–1. How are you, Al? [*Asking stereotyped question.*]

P–2. You know it hurts me to see an old man like that tied up in a strait jacket. Is it necessary to treat them like that?

N–3. It's not a matter of doing it for the heck of it, Al. Mr. ____ is very hyperactive, and by applying restraint it lessens the possibility of his hurting himself. You know he is watched fairly closely. Also you know he's very provoking and could get hurt by another patient, but being in a camisole he's less active and less provoking to the other patients. [*Giving an explanation. Defending.*]

P–4. If you untie him, I'll take care of him.

N–5. No, you better leave him tied. The aides know when to take him out. [*Refusing. Giving information.*]

P–6. You should have stuck around yesterday. I met with Dr. ____ and Dr. ____. They decided to send me downstairs for two weeks as a trial to see how I act and for a final decision on whether I can go home for the holidays. Dr. ____ said if everything works out well, I can go home.

N–7. I saw Drs. ____ and ____ come in to see Dr. ____ yesterday, but I didn't realize it was concerning you or I would have stopped to put in a good word. [*Giving information. Indicating willingness to be of assistance.*]

P–8. You know I was in this ward a short time ago, and I asked to go back upstairs.

N–9. Do you remember why? [*Requesting an explanation. Seeking meaning of the patient's action. Better worded, "What events led to your making this request?"*]

P–10. It's hard to remember, but the place was getting on my nerves. (Patient played with the ties of patient ____'s camisole.)

N–11. Would you feel better if we took him out and had him join us? [*The nurse is offering action designed to lessen the patient's anxiety.*]

P–12. Yes. It's very upsetting to see an old man like that tied up.

N–13. Can you tell me some other things that upset you, Al? [*Exploring. The nurse recognized the patient's use of the word "upsetting" and used it as a cue. The patient would not have had to answer as he did if he had been asked to tell the nurse some other kinds of things that have upset him* in the past. *The nurse might also have offered some explanation of why he asked the question; e.g., the nurse could say, "Perhaps it would be helpful if you and I spend some of our time together today to discuss the kinds of things that have tended to upset you before you came to the hospital." The nurse could have added, "I say this because many patients find that it helps to try to understand better the upsetting experiences they've had and their responses to them so that they can figure out what brought them to the point of becoming sick. Understanding this makes it less likely for you to become sick again."*]

P–14. Nothing really upsets me.

N–15. Did you get upset when your father was sick? [*The nurse has introduced a specific area for discussion rather abruptly—without explanation to the patient—and has taken the lead rather than leaving it to the patient.*]

P–16. I prayed for him to die. They refused to have him in the hospital as there was nothing they could do for him. The doctors said why prolong the inevitable. So I prayed for him to die. I was tempted to take a pillow and suffocate him. You must have seen people in the final stages of these illnesses.

N–17. Yes. It's not pleasant and particularly hard if it's one of your own family. . . . (Patient interrupted.) [*Accepting. The nurse is expressing his own feelings.*]

P–18. What would you do? Have you ever felt that way?

N–19. No. I feel sorry for the person and family, but what one does is make the person as comfortable as one can. [*Disagreeing. The patient* *was apparently looking for acceptance of his feelings. The nurse might have said, "No, but I can certainly see what you must have felt" and added, "In situations like that all we can do is try to make the person as comfortable as possible."*]

P–20. My father died of starvation. He took very little food and he looked it. I told you I was tempted to put that pillow over his face.

N–21. Would you say that seeing sick people upsets you? [*The patient repeats his feelings again, looking for acceptance. The nurse counters with a question. He might have preceded it with, "You wanted to end his suffering." The patient wants the nurse to understand that he felt helpless to help his father and wanted to ease his pain. He wants the nurse to let him know that he, the nurse, realizes that his "murderous thoughts" were not motivated by hostility.*]

P–22. Yes. When children get hurt, it also makes me feel bad. I'll talk to them and try and make them forget the pain.

N–23. Do things that happen at work upset you? [*The nurse has changed the subject somewhat and taken the lead. The patient is not given the opportunity to suggest other things that upset him.*]

P–24. If I catch somebody doping off on the job, especially after I treat them good, I'll read them out, and they seem to understand.

N–25. How do you act when this upsets you? [*Exploring. Encouraging description.*]

P–26. I curse them out.

N–27. Do you go any further? [*The nurse is being indirect and implies that more aggressive action occurs.*]

P–28. You mean hit him? No, I don't become abusive.

N–29. How do you think they feel when you're finished? [*The nurse seems to be indicating disapproval. The patient feels called on to justify his actions.*]

P–30. They probably curse me out, but they go back to work.

N–31. Have you ever gotten upset at your family? [*The nurse has introduced a new phase of the same general topic. However, the experiences introduced by the patient could have been discussed in much greater detail.*]

P–32. One time we were out drinking. My wife, brother, father, a friend, and myself. My wife was squawking to go home. I had too much to drink and slapped her with the back of my hand—not once, but about 10 times. This was about three years after I was married. I haven't touched her since that. I felt rotten and so ashamed. I felt as if I was the dirtiest _____ there was. Sometimes at the job when things get tough, I go out and get drunk.

N–33. Don't they miss you? [*Exploring. The patient may have profited from some response on the nurse's part to his feelings about hitting his wife. It might have helped if the nurse had said something like, "You felt badly when you lost control of yourself and hurt your wife." This might have led the patient to bring up other instances of his loss of control and the guilt that followed. The nurse misses a good opportunity to learn why he uses and sometimes overuses alcohol. The nurse might have said, "When things get too tough?" and explored what this meant.*]

P–34. No, I've never been caught.

N–35. Are you lucky? [*Suggesting tentative meaning.*]

P–36. No, I wouldn't exactly say that. You know they told my wife I was top man. My boss called my wife up and wanted to know when I was coming back to work. The business agent said I was looking swell and should get the hell out.

N–37. I think you're looking great also and should be ready to move on to another ward and then home. This will take time, as you well know, and patience as well. So we'll continue discussing whatever you like until the day you leave. [*Giving approval and encouragement. The nurse's last comment is most worthwhile.*]

P–38. I hope it's soon.

N–39. I must leave now. See you soon. [*Giving information.*]

P–40. Okay, Mr. L. So long.

This nurse-patient relationship was continued following the patient's transfer to an open ward. The patient was seen twice by the nurse during his stay on this new ward, during which time they discussed his plans for the future. He was discharged one week after his arrival on the open ward.

Contributors of Clinical Material

Janesy B. Myers, R.N., Chief Nurse, Veterans Administration Hospital, Northport, Long Island, New York

Mary M. Manley, R.N., Staff Nurse, Veterans Administration Hospital, Northport, Long Island, New York

Helen S. Moore, R.N., Supervisor, Veterans Administration Hospital, Northport, Long Island, New York

Clara Toscano Johns, R.N., Graduate of the Germantown Hospital, Philadelphia, Pennsylvania

Student nurses at the Albert Einstein Medical Center, Northern Division, Philadelphia, Pennsylvania

Student nurses at the School of Nursing, University of Pennsylvania, Philadelphia, Pennsylvania

Kenneth Larson, R.N.

Joyce Samhammer Hays, R.N.

Bibliography

Arieti, Silvano: "Schizophrenia: Other Aspects; Psychotherapy," *American Handbook of Psychiatry*. New York: Basic Books, 1959.

Bachand, Joan: *Problematic Verbal Patterns of Student Nurses in Initial Interviews with Psychiatric Patients: A Tool and Its Application*. Master's Thesis, College of Nursing, Rutgers–the State University of New Jersey, 1959.

Brammer, Lawrence M., and Everett L. Shostrom: *Therapeutic Psychology: Fundamentals of Counseling and Psychotherapy*. Englewood Cliffs, N.J.: Prentice-Hall, 1960.

Brown, Martha Montgomery, and Grace R. Fowler: *Psychodynamic Nursing*, 2nd ed. Philadelphia: Saunders, 1961.

Burton, Genevieve: *Personal, Impersonal, and Interpersonal Relations*. New York: Springer, 1958.

Fromm-Reichmann, Frieda: "Notes on the Development of Treatment of Schizophrenics by Psychoanalytical Psychiatry," *Psychiatry*, **2**:263–73, 1948.

———: *Principles of Intensive Psychotherapy*. Chicago: University of Chicago Press, 1950.

Hays, Joyce Samhammer: "Focusing on Feelings," *Nursing Outlook*, **10**:332–33, May 1962.

Karnosh, Louis J., and Dorothy Mereness: *Psychiatry for Nurses*, 5th ed. St. Louis: Mosby, 1958.

Matheney, Ruth V., and Mary Topalis: *Psychiatric Nursing*, 3rd ed. St. Louis: Mosby, 1961.

Peplau, Hildegard E.: *Interpersonal Relations in Nursing*. New York: Putnam's Sons, 1952.

———: "Talking with Patients," *Am. J. Nursing*, **60**:964–67, July 1960.

———: "Therapeutic Concepts," *Aspects of Psychiatric Nursing*. Section B. League Exchange, No. 26, National League for Nursing, 1957.

Rogers. Carl R.: "Characteristics of a Helping Relationship," *Personnel and Guidance Journal* (September 1958). Reprinted as Supplement No. 27, *Canada's Mental Health*, March 1962.

———: *Client-Centered Therapy*. Boston: Houghton Mifflin, 1951.

———: *Counseling and Psychotherapy*. Boston: Houghton Mifflin, 1942.

———: "A Counseling Approach to Human Problems," *Am. J. Nursing*, **56**:994–97, August 1956.

Schwartz, Morris S., and Emmy Lanning Shockley: *The Nurse and the Mental Patient.* New York: Russell Sage Foundation, 1956.

Sullivan, Harry Stack: *Conceptions of Modern Psychiatry,* 2nd ed. New York: Norton, 1953.

———: *The Psychiatric Interview.* New York: Norton, 1954.

WHO. *Expert Committee on Psychiatric Nursing. First report.* World Health Organization Technical Report Series, No. 105, July 1956.

Wolberg, Lewis R.: *The Technique of Psychotherapy.* New York: Grune and Stratton, 1954.

Index

Index

Accepting, 8, 21, 28, 89, 92, 109, 111, 125, 129, 187, 269, 270
Action, formulating plan of, 20, 23, 28, 130, 213
Advising, 28, 36, 75, 115, 196, 251
Agreeing, 8, 27, 36, 78, 190, 246, 251
Angry feelings, 12, 52, 55, 92, 96, 97, 190-91, 199, 208, 263-64
Anxiety, 1, 10, 11, 12, 14, 29, 114, 122, 171, 188-89, 190-92, 201, 225
Approval, 8, 9, 25, 27, 36, 53, 124, 149, 190, 191, 251, 257, 258, 260-61, 267, 271
Arieti, Silvano, 29
Autistic patient, 90-93, 99-102

Bachand, Joan, 36, 38
Belittling feelings expressed, 16, 32, 37, 117, 131, 132
Blame, 26, 145. *See also* Criticism; Disapproving
Brammer, Lawrence M., 7, 8, 13, 17, 20, 26, 27, 35
Brown, Martha Montgomery, 10, 19
Burton, Genevieve, 24, 25, 26, 28, 29, 30, 32

Capabilities, questioning, 30, 155, 239, 269
Challenging, 29, 36, 231, 242, 247
Clarification, 15, 22, 43, 45, 82, 91, 92, 95, 100, 127, 197, 238, 253
Clichés, 32, 146. *See also* Stereotyped comments
Closing the discussion, 20, 69, 72, 73, 86, 104, 118, 120, 202-3, 233, 242, 248, 265-66
Collaboration, 19, 23, 132, 169, 225, 228
Communication, 7, 8, 10, 11, 12, 13, 15, 17, 27, 35, 244, 248-49
Comparison, 11, 12, 21, 98, 101, 199, 252, 263
Conclusion, unwarranted, 179. *See also* Data, going beyond
Conditions, 9, 26, 198. *See also* Limits
Confidential nature of the relationship, 161, 186
Consensual validation, 16, 22, 27, 42, 43, 93, 107, 169, 206
Content, 18, 19, 42, 44
Criticism, 30. *See also* Blame; Disapproving

Data, gathering raw, 11, 27, 31, 45, 199
  going beyond, 201
  significance of, 20, 45, 172, 188, 200, 208
Defending, 27, 30, 37, 51, 82, 83, 125, 214, 239
Delusional ideas, 27, 29, 31, 33, 84, 234-36, 242, 243, 245
Denial, 34, 37, 78, 170, 242
Dependency, 41
Depression, 85, 139, 182-83. *See also* Suicidal ideas
Description of perceptions, 11, 21, 42, 80, 81, 96, 106, 133, 200, 205, 206, 217
Disagreeing, 27, 36, 51, 52, 79, 80, 237
Disapproving, 26, 36, 66, 74, 78, 80, 109, 118, 213, 239. *See also* Blame; Criticism
Distortions of reality, 16, 18, 29, 139, 157, 158, 180-81, 208, 215, 216-17, 225. *See also* Delusional ideas

Doubt, voicing, 16, 22, 42, 56, 97, 180-81, 255

Emotional illness, 1, 261
Evaluation, 2, 3, 18, 22, 27, 47, 48, 61, 66, 105, 115, 141, 212
Examples of interpersonal techniques, nontherapeutic, 36-37
therapeutic, 21-23
Explanation, requesting, 30, 37, 42, 46, 96, 100, 101, 105, 128, 230, 247
Exploring, 14, 22, 44, 92, 128, 133, 180, 250, 255, 271
External source, indicating existence of, 31, 37, 71, 79, 170, 231

Facial expression, 8, 34, 153, 197, 222, 232
Feelings, belittling, 16, 32, 37, 117, 131, 132
expression of, 8, 11, 13, 14, 19, 30, 52, 83, 84, 102, 128, 243, 259, 260, 263
mixed, 168-69
translating into, 18, 23, 45, 84, 88, 95, 99, 101
First hour of a relationship, 41, 65-69, 70, 90, 94, 99, 126, 229
Focusing, 14, 22, 138, 165, 171, 172, 206, 255
on minor detail, 140, 191, 230, 238
on nurse, 12, 66, 85, 110, 111, 120, 258
Formulation, of plan of action, 20, 23, 28, 130, 213
of meaning, 17, 18, 20, 46, 169, 188
Fowler, Grace R., 10, 19
Fromm-Reichmann, Frieda, 15, 25, 28, 34

Giving, 9, 201-2, 204

Hallucinations, 11, 128-37, 144, 148, 150, 172, 175, 176, 180, 181, 240
Hays, Joyce Samhammer, 18, 33
Helping role, 2, 147-48
Hostility. *See* Angry feelings
"How," 42, 44, 129, 252, 263, 265

Implied, verbalizing the, 17, 22, 43, 44, 97, 137, 142, 154, 204, 243, 247, 250
Information, giving, 14, 22, 28, 47, 98, 249, 252, 258
lack of, 42, 50, 242, 263
from clinical record, 65, 176, 254
Initiative, 7, 9, 35, 59, 62, 67, 73, 74, 104, 134, 165, 235-36, 249. *See also* Leading the discussion
Interpersonal role of the nurse, 2, 15, 19, 20, 69, 186, 199, 261-62
Interpersonal techniques, 1-37
Interpreting, 17, 34, 37, 46, 208
Interruptions, 182
Intimidating words, 31, 42, 43, 53, 117, 127, 169, 189, 193, 253

Karnosh, Louis J., 13

Leading the discussion, 9, 10, 140, 143, 269, 270. *See also* Initiative
Leads, general, 9, 21, 49, 152, 185, 197, 213, 214, 215, 219, 220, 259
Learning, 20, 25, 31, 35, 46, 199, 211, 221, 249
Limits, 3, 194, 198, 227, 233-34. *See also* Conditions
Literal responses, 33, 37, 54, 55, 62, 79, 87, 96, 99, 245

Matheney, Ruth V., 26, 35
"Mean," 53, 117, 127, 169, 189, 193
Meaning, formulation of, 17, 18, 20, 46, 169, 188. *See also* Significance of the data; Summarizing; Understanding
Medical patients, 121-25
Mereness, Dorothy, 13
Mood, 121, 138
Moralizing, 26, 145, 196
Mute patients, 11

Neurologic patient, 109-12
Nontherapeutic techniques, 2, 24-38
Nonverbal communication, 3, 7, 10, 12, 232

Notes, interaction, 15, 29, 46, 66, 160-61, 181
Nurse, focusing on, 12, 66, 85, 110, 111, 120, 258
  role of, 2, 15, 19, 20, 69, 186, 199, 261-62

Observations, making, 7, 10, 17, 21, 50, 98, 127, 203, 216, 217, 251
Obstetric patients, 113-118
Openings, broad, 9, 21, 41, 48, 49, 65, 90, 128

Patient's role, 9, 47, 59, 65, 67, 69
Patterns of interpersonal difficulties, recurring, 10, 12, 14, 152, 157, 167, 168-69, 180, 194, 199, 208
Pediatric patients, 103-8
Peplau, Hildegard E., 9, 11, 12, 15, 17, 18, 19, 25, 28, 31, 34, 45, 192
Perceptions, description of, 11, 21, 42, 80, 81, 96, 106, 133, 200, 205, 206, 217
Plan of action, formulating, 20, 23, 28, 130, 213
Praise, 25. *See also* Approval
Probing, 14, 28, 36, 89, 133, 134, 135, 140, 265
Problematic verbal patterns (Bachand), 36, 38
Process ("how"), 42, 44, 252, 263, 265

Reality, distortions of, 16, 18, 29, 139, 157, 158, 180-81, 208, 215, 216-17, 225
  presenting, 16, 22, 55, 59, 209, 222, 240, 254-55
Reassuring, 24, 36, 79, 130, 141, 145, 160, 184, 267, 268
Recognition, 8, 21, 71, 139, 258, 261
Reflecting, 13, 22, 48, 81, 88, 92, 100, 101, 105, 119, 124, 128, 134, 141, 225
Rejecting, 25, 36, 70, 73, 74, 75, 78, 182
Relationship, purpose of, 2, 15, 19, 20, 61, 69, 182-83, 248-49, 261-62
Restating, 12, 21, 43, 44, 45, 168, 206
Rogers, Carl R., 3, 8, 11, 12, 18, 19, 27, 28, 35
Role(s), of the nurse, 2, 15, 19, 20, 69, 186, 199, 261-62
  reversing, 66, 232
Role-playing, 20

Schwartz, Morris S., 7, 10, 12, 26, 33, 35
Self, offering, 9, 21, 45, 47, 48, 51, 52, 89, 115, 182
Sequence, placing event in, 10, 21, 85, 204, 206, 207, 210, 217, 218, 230
Shockley, Emmy Lanning, 7, 10, 12, 26, 33, 35
Shostrom, Everett L., 7, 8, 13, 17, 20, 26, 27, 35
Significance of the data, 20, 45, 172, 188, 200, 208. *See also* Formulation, of meaning; Summarizing; Understanding
Silence, 7, 9, 21, 48, 58, 59, 61, 62, 182, 199, 232, 258
Social relationship, 15, 67
Source, indicating existence of an external, 31, 37, 71, 79, 170, 231
Stereotyped comments, 9, 32, 37, 59, 76, 77, 117, 118, 236, 265. *See also* Clichés
Subject, changing the, 35, 66, 83, 88, 167, 231, 270. *See also* Unrelated topic
Suicidal ideas, 12, 70-89, 128, 136-47, 181, 200, 210. *See also* Depression
Sullivan, Harry Stack, 11, 15, 16, 17, 19, 24, 25, 30, 31, 32, 33, 35
Summarizing, 19, 23, 206-7, 210, 225, 226, 227, 265-66. *See also* Formulation, of meaning; Significance of the data; Understanding
Surgical patients, 117-20

Techniques, interpersonal, 1-37
Tentative meaning, suggesting, 63, 96, 97, 101, 202
Testing, 17, 29, 37, 74, 103, 104, 146, 230, 231, 236, 239, 240, 242, 249, 257
Themes. *See* Patterns of interpersonal difficulties, recurring
Therapeutic techniques, 2, 7-23

"They," 43, 144, 236, 245, 247, 250, 252
Time, placing event in, 10, 21, 107, 122, 145, 246
Topalis, Mary, 26, 35
Translating into feelings, 18, 23, 45, 84, 88, 95, 99, 101

Understanding, 8, 9, 11, 12, 14, 15, 16, 19, 27, 35, 45, 51, 169, 189, 203-4, 261, 269. *See also* Formulation, of meaning; Significance of the data; Summarizing
Unrealistic questions, 113, 130, 132, 243
Unrelated topic, 35, 37, 78, 79, 88, 133, 136, 142, 180, 232, 233. *See also* Subject, changing the

Validation, consensual, 16, 22, 27, 42, 43, 93, 107, 169, 206

"We," 41, 46, 173, 175, 257
"Why," 31, 42, 141, 190, 245
Wolberg, Lewis R., 9, 13, 14, 18, 20, 35
World Health Organization, 2